Life and Other Lies

John Wood

ISBN-10: 1460918541
ISBN-13: 978-1460918548

DEDICATION

To Suzanne, my solid ground in the quicksand of life.
To my three wonderful children,
John, Katie, and Kelsey.

CONTENTS

Introduction

There are parts of this story that are pretty ugly. Life just flat sucks sometimes. In fact, depending upon your definition of hell, life here on this planet can seem at times, like pure, unadulterated hell. Come to think of it, if you have experienced a life free from hellish encounters and you are into your fifties or sixties, you are an aberration. Sometimes even those who have not yet experienced a birthday are subjected to lives of loss and pain.

Why?

God only knows.

This is a story about loss. It is a story about pain. It is a story about the virtual shrapnel that rips us apart following a direct hit from one of the grenades of life. Sometimes it's an explosion of massive proportions. Sometimes it's little firecrackers that blow off pieces of our hearts over a period of years until one day we wake up and realize that we have a hole that has been slowly increasing in size for months or maybe even years.

There are also parts of this story that are wonderful and healing. Life at times can be beautiful. In fact, depending upon your definition of heaven, life here on this planet can seem like pure, unadulterated heaven at times. Come to think of it, if you have experienced a life free from wonderful, joyful encounters and you are into your fifties or sixties, you are an aberration.

This is a story about healing. It is a story about joy. It is a story about the sunlight from heaven that warms us and calms us and brings us at times, to a place of pure peace for which there is no explanation. Sometimes there are tiny raindrops of joy that fall almost imperceptibly, slowly refreshing and restoring our hearts until months or maybe even years later we experience the joy and the peace of healing.

If you long to experience this peace; if you long to experience this joy...stick around.

There are answers to the dichotomy between the seasons of heaven and the seasons of hell.

Stay tuned...

"Now it is required that those who have been given a trust must prove faithful." Paul, I Corinthians 4:2 NIV

"The requirements for a good guide are reliability and accurate knowledge. It matters very little to me what you think of me, even less where I rank in popular opinion. I don't even rank myself. I'm not aware of anything that would disqualify me from being a good guide for you, but that doesn't mean much. God makes that judgment." Paul, I Corinthians 4:3-5 The Message

I believe that the events in the life of my wife Suzanne and I, inclusive of my daughter's death are a trust given to us by God. This project is a feeble attempt to prove faithful to that God-given trust. It is far beyond "not easy" to recall and document events that occurred during a period of life that was filled with hurt, loss, tremendous pain, and fractured faith. One thing that remains crystal clear in my understanding however, is that God never once promised otherwise. One reason that God has given us this trust I believe, is to somehow convey that the hurt, the pain, and the loss are not the end of the story, they are the beginning. You can trust us on this. If it weren't so, we would have given up long ago.

Oh, and one more thing...

"I was unsure about how to go about this, and felt totally inadequate - I was scared to death, if you want the truth of it - and so nothing I said could have impressed you or anyone else. But the message came through anyway. God's Spirit and God's power did it..."   Paul, I Corinthians 2 The Message

Prologue

I hope you stay with me here. We are beginning in a place that may be a bit uncomfortable for some. You may or may not be a believer. You may believe in God. You may even believe in Jesus as the son of God; God come to earth in human form. Now we are beginning to stretch the belief however. Yes, I believe in God you may say, and yes, I believe in Jesus. It is difficult however, to get my head around the concept of Jesus as the essence of God made human; Jesus becoming flesh and blood; to believe that Jesus was and continues to be real; and the Holy Spirit? Well now, that really is a stretch. How in the world do I get my head around that one? The Spirit of God sent to counsel and comfort, when I can't see or hear him? Consider me if you will, as a fellow traveler who has come to and passed the fork in the road. You remember don't you; the solitary road that branches into two, requiring us to make a life altering choice; requiring us to choose which to travel with minimal information about each?

I have at times, entertained some substantial questions about the road that I have chosen. I have even been inclined to "unchoose" the one I'm on and to laboriously cut a trail to the other one. Let me get some things out of the way right up front before exploring the road that I have chosen. I find what religion often represents to be highly offensive in many cases. More people have likely been murdered in the name of religion and in religious wars than in all of the other great wars combined. I know that I am walking a fine line here.

Have I offended those of you who grew up in "church" and hold firmly and rightly in many cases to doctrines passed down for generations? If we are to deal openly and effectively with loss and grief, my firm belief is that we must question and test in our quest to obtain real answers in the midst of tremendous pain, and colossal doubt about the true nature of a God who would allow these horrible things to happen to us. A God who watches us suffer unbelievable pain as we witness a ghastly, and life altering train wreck; a catastrophic event as it were, that brutalizes and kills a loved one, and sucks the very life out of us when it happens. How could a God who apparently sits comfortably in heaven watching all of these horrendous events unfold, be the God that He says He is in the Bible? Is there even an answer, and if so does the answer even matter?

Maybe God can shed some light...

John, have you ever seen a lioness protect her cubs? Have you ever seen a woman protect her children? Fierce John, very fierce; and believe me, as much of a warrior as you are, I assure you that you do not want any part of that action. John you were born into a world at war. The strongman saw to that. I do have an ultimate plan here however, one that I have had since I created the universe. But I can see by the look on your face that you don't get it yet. John, John, John, you try my patience! Fortunately for you and the rest of mankind, my patience is infinite and eternal.

Otherwise you would now be toast.

But I digress. As a result of that ultimately ferocious heavenly battle a course was set that must be completed. Once the strongman was defeated, he was cast out of my home and sent to live in yours. Yes, yes, I know it doesn't make sense to you yet, but just stay with me here. You see John; the strongman was not

the only one cast out of my home. All of the traitorous angels who fought alongside him were run out of town as well. And where do you think they were all booted to John? They are all right there with you...for now. Remember, I said earlier that there is a master plan in place here that has not yet been completed. War is hell. Life on this earth can sometimes seem like a small taste of hell. The end result, the completion as it were, is eternal punishment for some, angels and humans alike, and

eternal joy for others. But until then...

LIFE AND OTHER LIES

To whom do you turn, where do you go, and how do you cope when tragedy and loss make a train wreck of your life? This is not a five step plan for recovery. It is not a formula. It is one family's story. The answers begin with the hot and caustic pain that flows from the cauldron of loss. They continue as what was once hot and caustic becomes cooler and begins to slowly lose its sting.

I can assure you that regardless of what you have lost and the state of your spiritual and emotional life, there is beauty to be found in your pain. This is a place for those who have experienced loss; loss of any kind. During the course of our lives we will all experience loss of some sort. Whether it is a job, a spouse, a marriage, a child or any other number of things that can disappear in the blink of an eye. In my case it has been a job, very nearly a marriage, and most profoundly the loss of a precious child. The repercussions were enormous. I came dangerously close to personally destroying a marriage, and accepting a lifetime of grief. By the grace of God, and my wife's great love and patience, my marriage survived and though the grief has never completely vanished, it has become a more manageable piece of my new life without my daughter Kelsey. We will discuss the journey back to joy. No it will never be the same again. I am sure that this is the most difficult

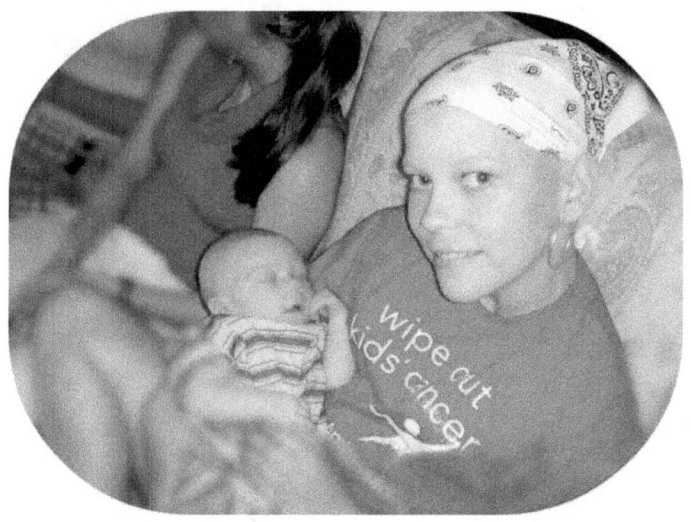

factor in loss to accept. We want our old lives back. We want things to be the same as they were before. But they can't be. However, we can begin creating a new life beginning right here, right now, regardless of our point of reference. We will cry, we will laugh, and most of all we will work together to find meaning and healing in the losses that we have experience

1

WINNOWING

In the grand scheme of life, five or ten years seems a small block of time. In the grand scheme of eternity, a life seems exceedingly minute in duration. And indeed it is, if we choose to believe what God has to say about life, death, and life again. If you maintain a different perspective however, I encourage you to read our story and participate with us in this journey regardless of your current frame of reference. I sincerely believe that we will both benefit from the association. I do not now know or profess to ever take hold of understanding the mind of God. Job's understanding was far beyond mine when he responded to God, *"Surely I spoke of things too wonderful for me to know."* God is far beyond my feeble ability to fully comprehend. Even the concept of God leaves me grasping for understanding. You will encounter ample evidence of this as we begin this journey together. Before we begin our association however, I feel compelled to share with you two events that, though they happened to me, resonate still today with profound impact on my entire family. We lived them together. They should serve as enlightening antecedents to the refining events that follow them. There is a great deal of pain in the story that you have chosen to read, but if you will momentarily indulge me, we will eventually travel to a place of great beauty.

In the fall of 1993, my family and I were in Baton Rouge, Louisiana where I was managing a branch location for a national chain of retail "off price" stores. I was in a word, miserable. My fortieth birthday loomed large on the horizon, and I was completely depleted physically, spiritually, and emotionally. My wife Suzanne was just beginning her encounter with what we would later come to know as panic disorder. My two oldest children John and Katie had attended three different schools in the past twelve

months, and I was under tremendous pressure at work to turn around a severely struggling retail operation. I was working twelve to sixteen hours a day and collapsing when I arrived at home, with no additional time or energy to invest in my family. There were bright spots of course. On my one day off each week, the two oldest children and I would spend at least an hour or so at a local park. These were cherished times that remain so in my memory even today.

In early February of nineteen ninety-four, I flew from Baton Rouge to San Antonio, Texas for a meeting to discuss severe cut backs and a corporate reorganization. The meeting was difficult and stressful, consisting primarily of upper management clearly defining the shortcomings of those of us in middle management. I flew out of San Antonio at seven that evening stopping at DFW airport in Dallas Fort Worth for a connecting flight into Baton Rouge. The flight from DFW to Baton Rouge had us on a small American Eagle commuter plane for a rough but uneventful ride. My mind was occupied with thoughts of home and tomorrow's activities. I knew that once again I would return home late in the evening after my children were in bed and rise early the next morning for another long day. Somewhere in the midst of my quiet thoughts of home and rest, the plane suddenly began to bounce and buck like a bull in the rodeo. I chalked it up initially to incredibly rough weather, and held on for what I thought would be a brief ride. This first ride was brief but unfortunately only the beginning of the rodeo. There was much more to come. As I glanced out the left side window, I was alarmed to see red and yellow flames flaring from the small turbo prop engine. Subsequently, I heard a clicking sound as something began to pelt the side of the plane. My initial thoughts were not of fear, but of expectation that the plane could certainly land with a single engine. These thoughts were immediately interrupted by a fellow passenger's gasp from the right side seating area. I glanced over at her side of the plane to discover that the right side turbo-prop was throwing off the same red and yellow flames. No sooner had I seen the flames than they stopped, apparently almost simultaneously, with the flames from the left side engine. At this point the plane became incredibly silent and dark save for the flashing emergency light at the back of the cabin. I vaguely remember the sick roller coaster feeling as the plane plunged nose down from twelve thousand feet towards the darkness below. The minutes immediately following were filled with thoughts bathed in rationalization. I continued to rationalize that things were not as bad as they seemed. I believed that we would eventually find the lights of the runway and land powerless but safely. Strikingly, the cabin continued to remain ominously silent with no word from the pilot or the flight attendant who along with the rest of us, continued to remain buckled in and clueless. At some point, through the capable hands of a former Vietnam War pilot, our "spiral towards the ground" as a witness described it, somehow became a glide. As the plane leveled and floated through the darkness I began to look for the airport out my window. I began to ask God repeatedly to glide us just a little closer, much as if we had run out of gas in our car and were trying to coast to the nearest gas station. Amazingly, there was not the slightest hint of a human voice on the airplane with every passenger praying silently and focused on the harsh reality of what lay ahead for the small plane falling out of the Louisiana sky. I continued to ask God to get us just a little further towards the airport so that we could find a runway to come down on. For what seemed like an eternity, I strained to see the ground below us, hoping to spot a runway amidst the sporadic lights, trees, and open fields. I remember seeing the lights of Baton Rouge in the distance, and thinking that if we could just make it to the lights of the runway, we would live. Suddenly and without warning my thoughts were interrupted as the body of the plane violently met the ground below us. I immediately felt thankfulness even as the plane bounced wildly past a concrete embankment to our left, hit a metal fence and sailed over a forty-foot concrete ditch to the other side (carrying the fence with us). We eventually came to rest within feet of a major roadway. I heard the pilot warn the flight attendant of a fuel leak, and together they began frantically moving passengers down the aisle and off the plane. I distinctly remember being the last passenger off the plane followed by the flight attendant and captain. I jumped through the side door exit and sunk down into the mud of a soggy, cut over sugar cane field.

Fast-forward to June of 1994, to an inner city classroom of severely autistic nine to fourteen year olds. I am doing everything I can to cajole a young lady from continuing to pick at an open sore on her leg that holds endless fascination in her autistic world. I am unsuccessful and the sore begins to bleed even as she continues to "stim" on it. Fortunately it is time for outside activities and her attention is finally pulled elsewhere. My week in an autistic classroom is one of several that I will spend during the summer of 1994 as I prepare for my new role, job, responsibility, occupation, and ultimately life as a special education teacher in the Dallas ISD. By mid-August, I will be standing in a classroom of fourteen seven to twelve year old severely emotionally disturbed children having exhausted what I thought would be a full day of lessons in approximately an hour and a half. How I survived my first day is no longer a mystery. The grace of God is the only phrase that is applicable. There is no other explanation. To survive not only my first day, but also an additional three years of daily life with an assortment of classroom occupants from environments filled with horrendous physical, emotional and sexual abuse is attributable only to the grace, hope, love and guidance of an all-knowing and loving Holy Father. To begin the journey even as I wrestled with my own emotional demon of post traumatic stress disorder is even more clearly a matter of divine intervention. There were days when I wondered not only how I could continue to cope with their needs, but how I could survive the day with my own sanity intact. There were many days that the post traumatic stress would trigger anxiety or panic in me even as I wrestled with children haunted by their own emotional demons. Though I did not always recognize it at the time, I can now clearly see the gentle hand of the Father as he worked with my hurts, pains and inadequacies to gently grow me spiritually so that I could in some small way, provide hope and direction for my constantly changing, rag tag band of students.

There were angels brought by the father to guide and direct me on a daily basis. Once again, it is only by looking back with the wisdom gained since; that I am able to recognize the Father's hand in what was at the time a terribly broken life. I now recognize not only my own brokenness, but also the tremendous brokenness of the students so generously entrusted to my often incompetent care. We came to know and love each other through our own weaknesses, our own pain, our own hurts that sometimes threatened to overwhelm us and steal what little joy there seemed to be in each day. Though the joy was small at first, as I began to recognize and rely on God a little more each day, the joy began to grow, and the pain, which had at one time been all consuming, began to recede. As my own pain began to abate, my ability to provide spiritual and emotional nourishment for my students began to increase. Some of them, though we are years beyond our most recent time together, continue to occupy a cherished place in my heart. Not because our times together were exceedingly joyful and wonderful. They certainly were anything but. No, it is because they were not times of great joy, but times of great trial, difficulty and anger that they hold such a special place in my thoughts. The love born of these relationships was one of hard work and deliberate action even in the face of constant anger and attack. I was forced to confront young children who had been so abused by the adults in their lives, that the only interaction they understood was fear, anger and physical violence. Though they cursed me, spat on me, bit me, kicked me, threw desks and books at me, and screamed at me, I intuitively understood that to reciprocate in kind would only exacerbate the pain in their already wounded hearts. How much of this and infinitely more, was done to Jesus on his journey to the cross? How much do we do to hurt Him daily when we reject his teaching and act in ways contrary to His will? When we ignore him and become absorbed in things of this life and this world that hold no permanent value, we cause him great pain. And Jesus reacts to this pain with a deliberate show of love. How could I not deliberately love the broken children entrusted to my care? How could I not love the seemingly unlovable? Those who by nature violate every long held tenet of decency that we have been taught to hold dear and even holy? Indeed, it violates my human nature to love those in this condition. It flies in the face of what I feel for them which is in many cases revulsion. To make physical contact with a child who has not bathed for days, and carries the resulting stench on his body, who has cursed you, screamed at you, and spit on you only moments before, is an act of will that violates basic human nature. It is more than an act of will it is an act of love. As my first year progressed with this rag tag bunch of castoffs, I continued to learn and grow in what seemed to be sporadic fits in the midst of constant stress and turmoil.

What I learned, but did not fully comprehend at the time, was the joy that exists in spite of extreme difficulty and turmoil. Even though I am now separated by job, time and distance from those incredibly battered and needy children, I continue to think about them and wonder from time to time what has happened in their lives since we separated. There is a loving place in my heart that will always exist for them, and I pray that they are happy, healthy and safe in their current circumstance. My time with them was difficult but well spent as preparation for the next incredibly complex, frightening, and challenging chapter in our family's story.

2

SHOCK

Our story of cancer begins in 1999, when my youngest daughter Kelsey was diagnosed with Ewing's Sarcoma. This disease is relatively rare with approximately one hundred fifty individuals, primarily children, receiving a diagnosis each year. As many who are reading will understand, the pain of diagnosis is overwhelming. I remember clearly, standing in the examining room waiting for the specialist to return and having a terrible feeling of impending disaster. It is a feeling I will never forget. A young doctor who had examined Kelsey following the specialist's examination, soon returned to the room and asked us to meet with the specialist in the x-ray room. The following events are forever etched in my memory. The specialist, a surgeon by training, was brutal in his communication with us. He felt certain that it was cancer, and most likely one of two kinds of bone cancer. He suggested that we schedule a biopsy quickly and begin treatment as soon as the results were in. As I sat listening, I felt an incredible urge to be somewhere, anywhere, other than where we were. I wanted desperately to wake up and find that it had been a bad dream, even as I knew intellectually that it could not and would not be. The next words I recall were instructions to move to the x-ray room for lung x-rays before leaving. I became desperate for relief, knowing without being told that the x-rays were to discover if the cancer had already metastasized to Kelsey's lungs. In my weakness, I could bear no more and walked in a stupor from the examining area to the waiting room. After sitting briefly in the waiting room I made my way to the men's room to throw up, leaving my wife Suzanne to handle the situation at hand alone.

The lung x-rays were negative, praise God, and Suzanne, Kelsey and I soon left the hospital in a fog. Kelsey had recently celebrated her ninth birthday, and would mature quickly in the days to come. As I write and relive Kelsey's diagnosis, I am reminded that so many others have experienced their own unique version of the events that I have described. None I am sure have been any easier or less overwhelming than our own. My father, who is now in perfect peace in heaven, had been diagnosed with advanced prostate cancer in 1994. His diagnosis was unexpected and difficult. It was not however, as devastating as having my youngest child diagnosed five years later.

Until my father was diagnosed with cancer in 1994, our immediate family had been blessed with very little serious illness. I did understand and thank God for this often, having at the time the feeling that it couldn't last. My father worked hard for his family and for retirement, maintaining a high level of frugality when he could easily have afforded to spend more. I thought it ironic and distressing that after working so hard and denying himself for so many years, that at the beginning of retirement he should find that he probably would not live to enjoy the fruits of his labor. My father immediately made an appointment to see one of the most respected urologists in Texas to discuss his situation. He was told that surgery was not an option and that he should go home and enjoy as much as possible the remaining months of his life. That was nine years before he left us. Obviously he chose not to follow the doctor's recommendation. He was there for us following Kelsey's diagnosis even as his own treatment progressed. He provided unwavering support for us and for her until he became physically unable to leave his home. I prayed for my father's healing, but I did not truly believe that God would provide for it.

Over the course of Kelsey's illness and recurrence, I have seen several children die as a result of this rotten disease. Why have some survived while others have not? Why do beautiful, sweet children, in some cases infants, suffer with this disease when they obviously have done nothing themselves to deserve it? Does God want these children to die? Does he cause them to die? Is it for his glory or some other reason apparent only to him that they are allowed to leave us prematurely? Even if God does not cause this illness, he certainly allows it to be visited upon some and not others. Why? Short of death, why are some allowed to suffer terrible pain and indignity (hair loss, severe weight gain or loss, constant nausea, mouth sores etc.) as a result of the illness? I do not profess to take ownership of the answers to these questions, but I do wish to walk with you through our shared suffering. If you will continue with me through this process, I believe that God holds great benefit in store for us. It may not yet be clear, and there may currently be more questions in your mind than answers, but we will indeed benefit. Though your faith in God may have been shaken to its core, and your life may have been rocked with difficulty and pain, please give it a chance and stay with me through the following pages. Knowing as you do, that I am one who continues to suffer and question right along with you, please know as well, that in spite of the free fall of suffering we experience, we will surely land softly on the ground that God has prepared.

One more thing... well two really. You will notice that I change syntax and begin the next section writing as if speaking to my daughter Kelsey. I will shift between present and past tense as well. Please once again, bear with me in this indulgence. It fits perfectly my frame of mind and reference for this period in the journey. Please know as well, that I am simply the scribe for what is very much a family story. We lived it together.

3

ILLNESS JOURNAL

November 19th, nineteen ninety-nine. A huge swelling on the top of your shoulder blade. To the emergency room at eight, at home at two-thirty the following morning. No indication of what the problem was. Probably an injury the doctors said. November 22nd, a visit to your pediatrician and another visit to the orthopedic guy with an MRI scheduled for the next day. November 23rd, the orthopedic guy calls to say that it "appears" to be a hematoma. He says to give it a couple of weeks to disappear. We have some feeling of relief, but never expected it to be anything major anyway. Great Thanksgiving! You were fine and never seemed to notice the swelling, but I did. It bothered me some, but not much. Back to work on Monday. Normal day, nothing happening out of the ordinary. November 30th, Suzanne calls at work to tell me that the orthopedic guy called. He had sent the MRI to a tumor specialist. The tumor specialist wants to see you as quickly as possible. Ok, no need to panic, we'll take it one step at a time. Still, probably nothing serious. The doctors are just being cautious.

December 2nd, I read a magazine while we wait to see the tumor specialist. Your grandmother shows up and brings you a present. Time to see the doctor. We enter the examination room and begin our wait for the doctor. I read a magazine then put it down to pray. I ask God to let there be nothing seriously wrong with you. A nice young man, a "fellow" doing specialized training with the tumor specialist comes in to examine you. No swollen lymph nodes, everything seems ok. I breathe a small sigh of relief. He leaves and returns with the tumor specialist, a very matter of fact man with a direct approach. This is the first indication we have that this may be something serious, and it comes quickly. He tells us that you definitely have a tumor, and that he will meet us in the x-ray room to discuss the specifics of how we will proceed. I feel an instant flush in my face. My pulse begins to quicken. I stand and face the counter, lean over and grab it with my hands. I take a deep breath and begin to pray. It does not get better. We are taken to the x-ray room where we wait for about five minutes before the doctor arrives. My mind will not accept what I know is coming. I cringe when the doctor begins to speak. I don't want to hear this! He points to the x-rays, shows us a place on your scapula, and tells us that this is the tumor and that it could be malignant or benign, but that it is most probably malignant. I forget to breathe. My mind is numb. We will not know for sure until they do a biopsy. He tells us that the indicators say that it is an osteosarcoma, which is a form of bone cancer. I breathe deeply, somehow unable to accept this diagnosis. They want to x-ray your lungs. This can't be happening. I have to leave. I must get out of this room! I flee to the waiting room and tell your grandmother. She begins to speak, but I have no idea what she is saying. It is more than I can handle trying to process what I have just heard. In a couple of minutes I get up and go to the men's room. I grab the sink and hold on tightly. I quietly begin to cry. This is only the beginning Kelsey, of the times that your mother will be there for you during the hours, minutes and days that you need her most. Though I left the room, she remained. When I went to work, she remained. Whether spending day after day with you in the hospital or putting her own needs aside while you are at home, she will become the glue that binds us together as a family during this crisis. On this day, I eventually realize that there is no place else to go, and return to the doctor's office. However, I can't bring myself to go back into the treatment room. They are doing your chest x-ray to make sure it has not spread.

No God,

I don't want to know!

I don't want to know!

Thus began our journey. I did learn that day, that there was no indication that the disease had spread to your lungs. That was good news. You went the same week for a bone scan, a lung scan and a general CT scan. It was difficult waiting for those results as well, but nothing unusual was found on these reports. Each time we are forced to be in the surgeon's office, I get a horrible sick feeling. I have a terrible fear that someone will walk in and tell us that the cancer has spread or some other devastating news. I am just beginning to take the first steps toward turning this over to God. It is only now beginning to slowly tease my thought process that I am not in control of this situation. Something terrible is happening to you Kelsey, and there is nothing that I can do about it. I continually pray for strength. You have been such a trooper so far. You have done things that I know have been very foreign and frightening for you, but you have done them bravely and willingly. You have such trust in us when we tell you everything will be ok. I only wish that my belief were as strong as yours.

Friday of this same week brings us to your biopsy. There have been test and visits to the doctor and the hospital in between. You continue to be an inspiration to me with your strength and trust. Your mother is an equal inspiration. Without exception, she has been by your side throughout this entire process. Through each test, each discussion with the doctors, and each round of disheartening news. When I had to leave the room, because I just couldn't bear it any longer, she remained, held your hand, and heard the news that neither of us wanted to hear. While I was crying and being sick in the bathroom, she was there with you, hurting inside beyond description, but maintaining an exterior of strength for you. It is biopsy day and a great many of our friends and loved ones are present. You are at your best, holding court and laughing even though I know you are nervous. It's not until thirty minutes prior to surgery, after receiving medication that has lowered your resistance and inhibitions that the anxiety begins to show. We follow you down the long hallway and into the elevator. You have a death grip on your mother's hand, quietly crying as we proceed. Once in the hallway leading to surgery, you grab her hand even tighter and cry for her not to let you go. But she must. As you roll the few feet further toward surgery, leaving us behind, your cries become louder as your mother's pain increases with the rising level of your voice. Once your bed is through the door, your mother and I turn quietly to walk away, and for the first time she is visibly shaken. She immediately begins to sob, as we look for a hidden corner to collect our emotions. Your mother grabs my shoulders and collapses in my arms immersed in deep and painful cries of the heart. She vows never again to allow you to be taken away from her in that manner.

I am sitting in the chapel with about thirty or forty wonderfully supportive family and friends. All I want is time and space to pray. As I find a spot on a back pew, a dear friend sits beside me and takes my hand. We both pray silently and fervently. I will never forget this time with these wonderful people. Nor will I soon forget my time of prayer with this sensitive and Godly man. He and I both plead silently with God on your behalf. In a moment of intense care and support, another trusted friend literally falls to his knees in the hospital hallway in front of doctors and nurses pleading in your behalf Kelsey. These are only two of so many others who are openly and fervently asking God for mercy, and offering their heartfelt support. I pray for God to allow the biopsy to be negative. Oh, how I will shout and praise him if this is so! I reach a point in prayer when I feel comfortable with God. I don't know what his plan for us is, but I will accept his plan. I am comfortable with ending my prayer. I move to the hallway outside the chapel, and wait. Within fifteen minutes, I glance down the hallway and see the surgeon walking toward us. Once again, I want to run and not hear the news, but instead I quickly enter the chapel and tell your mother that it is time. She meets me outside as the doctor arrives. My hand is around her shoulder and hers around my waist as the doctor tells us that you definitely have a sarcoma. I begin to shake, but I listen, and ask questions. Without God's help and my earlier prayer conversation with him I would not have had peace with this process. The news is not the best that we had hoped for, nor is it what I had prayed so fervently for just minutes before. There is calmness and a peace however, that surrounds me, and in the heat of this moment I have a comfort that I can't describe. God gives me the strength somehow to communicate your situation to the beautiful and caring group who have assembled and prayed with us during your surgery. I am overwhelmed with the impact of this situation, but God is beginning to work with me. It will be a matter of days however, before my peace is shattered.

4

FREEFALL

It is Wednesday of the week following your biopsy. We continue to wait for the biopsy results. At work I am able to involve myself with the things that I enjoy most. You have been in my thoughts however, for the better part of the day. I continue to pray that your cancer will be an Osteosarcoma. If you must have cancer I would prefer that God allow you to have the more treatable kind, the one with the better survival rate. That has been my fervent prayer throughout most of the day. About four-thirty the phone rings and your mother is on the other end. The only words that I remember hearing are "it's Ewings". I immediately feel a weight begin to press on my head. It descends to my shoulders and into my torso and legs. I feel like I must weigh three hundred pounds. Once again I am numb. Earlier I had prayed that God would allow your biopsy to show no cancer. I had envisioned the doctor coming out in disbelief to let us know that he had been mistaken; there was no cancer after all. In my fantasy, I then let the doctor know that I had believed that this would be the case all along. God had answered our prayers in a mighty way, and Mr. surgeon, you had better understand that God is responsible for this miracle in spite of your disbelief.

It did not happen.

It was cancer.

My next immediate thought was along the lines of "yes its cancer, but it's very treatable, particularly the Osteosarcoma that the surgeon truly believes that you have". "It's Ewings". Oh please! How could God not answer this prayer? I was not happy about the cancer thing God, but okay, it was something that I could deal with if I had to. This however, is bad news upon previous bad news. Come on God, I need some good news! This is not what I was desperately praying for! I hang up the phone and immediately turn my chair away from my desk to avoid the gaze of anyone passing in the hall. I really do not know what to think at this point. I am stunned and unable to focus. I begin to pray. Prayer calms me and I begin to look for rays of hope in this unwanted news. I am beyond the ability to focus any longer at work, so I quietly leave. I really don't feel like talking to anyone about it right now.

Once at home my spirit begins to rise, and I decide to go for a run. At the track there is a young girl with her dad. She begins to chase her dog around the track, laughing with delight as she calls his name. I look at them with a bit of envy and more than a little sadness. How many opportunities have I missed with you Kelsey? How many hours have I not spent with you that I have instead spent in my own solitary pursuits? Will I even have another opportunity to spend time with you this way? The remainder of my run is spent with these thoughts and I feel an unfamiliar sadness as I drive home. Once at home I begin to feel somewhat better, and greet your mother cheerfully as she arrives home. As I turn to see her face I am immediately frightened. She is ashen. I ask what's wrong and she raises her hand to indicate that she is unable to talk about it at this point. It has been a cold evening and I have already removed my sweaty shirt to keep my body from chilling. As we arrive in the bedroom I ask her again to tell me what is going on. She is fighting back tears as she relays to me that the oncologist has just called to let us know that you will need a bone marrow test. He indicates that this is standard procedure with Ewing's sarcoma because there is a tendency for it to spread to this area. By this point I am visibly shaking. I literally crawl onto the bed on my hands and knees and maintain this position as I seek to absorb this new information. I am still shaking as I slowly begin to chant "no, no, no". It is almost subconscious at this point. Eventually your mother leaves the room and I begin to sob and shake uncontrollably. I fall from the bed to the floor on my hands and knees, and begin to pray. This is the only time Kelsey, that I remember asking God why.

There are three words that stay with me from that conversation. They are

please, **no** and **why**.

Beyond pleading with God for your life, I can only remember repeating them over and over as if they were a mantra. Later the same evening, you are alone with your mother and ask her directly and pointedly if you will die as the result of this illness. In her wisdom she tells you that we will all die at our own appointed time, but that we are going to do everything we can to beat this cancer and keep you with us for many years to come. This is also an opportunity to call your brother and sister together with us to explain your situation to them. We tell them that people with cancer sometimes die, but that we will continue to pray and seek treatment that will preserve your life here with us. We pray holding hands and gain strength from each other.

At the clinic on Friday, I am visibly weak. Your mother and I sit in the examining room with you while we wait for the doctor to arrive. This is all so new, and I am so afraid of hearing more bad news. I have a terrible fear that every visit with a doctor will bring more news that I don't want to hear. That is why I sit waiting but not minding the wait. It is certainly preferable to having someone come in and once again shatter what hope I have left. The first to visit us is an oncology "fellow". He seems very nice. He speaks to you, and treats you kindly, even though the examination is painful. He even gets you to laugh just a little. He leaves and we return with you to the waiting room. As everyone else sits, I stand and stare. It is the best way for me to pray in this setting. It just seems to be so difficult to find the right place and moment to pray in the middle of all the commotion of the hospital. I have a tendency to pray intensely; focusing solely on the prayer and tuning everyone, and everything else out. I am able to do this briefly today. As I stand and pray, I see the oncologist round the corner and approach us. We exchange greetings and he leads us into another examining room while you stay with your granny and papa. Your oncologist is a very kind man who spends at least forty five minutes with us describing the protocol that will be used to fight your cancer. He uses a great deal of medical terminology that is new to us now, but will become all too familiar as the weeks and months pass. And all of these new people; the doctors, nurses, technicians, therapist and many others; they will all become not only more familiar, but in many cases good and trusted friends.

Your oncologist informs us that you will be admitted to the hospital immediately and that your chemotherapy will begin tomorrow. He gently reminds us that you will quickly lose your hair. He adds that your bone marrow test will be done today before you are admitted. He then leaves and we return to prepare you for the hair loss. Amazingly, this seems to be of greater concern to you than the cancer itself. I will later come to understand that losing your hair is something that put you on display among your friends and leads you to desperately want to return to the life of "fitting in" that you have left behind. I will also weep at times as I long for the life that has been irretrievably lost for all of us. The longing for that life becomes an ache in my heart as you speak of the classmate who publicly ridiculed you as "Kelsey the bald headed bitch." However, on this day, God has seen fit to leave me clueless to the pain that awaits, as the nurses prepare you for the coming bone marrow test. You are moved to another room and given a drug designed to render you oblivious to the painful testing. It does its work as intended but also leaves you hallucinating bugs on the ceiling of the treatment room. As you climb onto the table the nurses move you face down on the table and ask you to relax. As they prepare the equipment, I see a large needle with a circumference that is greater than any I have seen to date. The nurse then buries the six inch long needle into your back until it reaches, then passes into your hip bone. Even though you are heavily sedated, you moan and squirm on the table as the same procedure is performed on both hips leaving holes as the needles are removed. It is my first taste of witnessing your pain and feeling helpless to relieve it. Even more so than the physical pain is the emotional and psychic pain that will follow you throughout your treatment and will leave me hurting and powerless to remove. Tears that begin here this day become my frequent companion in the months to come.

It is now New Year's Eve nineteen ninety-nine and your mother and I sit together in your hospital room as you receive the poisonous drugs that we pray will kill your cancer before it kills you. You are asleep as we mindlessly sit and repeatedly replay "welcome to the year two thousand" as spoken by a new year's celebrating doll given to us by friends. This is now your third round of chemo, and your hair is almost completely gone. My heart aches as I recall the tears you shed as you sat in the middle of the den floor and discovered that you were now able to easily remove large clumps of hair with your hands. Your face was in your hands and your back arched with each sob. I wanted so badly to ease your nine year old pain Kelsey, but I was once again powerless to do so. As we sat in your room that evening you mercifully slept. You have not eaten in three days, which we find becomes a regular part of your chemotherapy outcome. Your mother and I are now beginning to realize the full impact of this situation that we are in. I believe now, that you knew from the beginning Kelsey; probably even before your mother and I. This is only the beginning of the new life that will become all too familiar as we travel this road together. Your mother and I will spend countless days and nights in the hospital room with you as you endure what will become a five and one half year nightmare of treatment and remission. Your brother and sister, who are just now beginning their junior high school years, will soon come to understand that your mother and I will only sporadically be available to them as parents. It is not by design, but is in our minds, the only logical option. We cannot leave you alone and frightened in the hospital as you receive treatment that precipitates extreme nausea and vomiting as well as horrible and painful sores in your mouth and throat. It is a treatment that will weaken you and lower your resistance to the point that we will spend many nights in the emergency room waiting for you to admitted because your body is weak and feverish from the poison in your system. Later we will realize that the consequences of treatment will also leave you with irreversible lung damage and heart issues as well. As we move forward in your treatment the days begin to merge and at times become indistinguishable one from the other. I am sure it is the same for you. I have the easiest job. I get up and go to work in the morning, and visit you and your mother in the hospital in the evening. On the weekends I am able to spend most of the day there with you as many of our wonderful friends continue to visit through the weeks that move into months. During the course of your lengthy stays on the "cancer floor", we will watch many other children come and go. Some will simply leave the hospital when they finish treatment but others will leave to be remembered by a eulogy and a gravestone. It is not something that is explicitly stated when we ask the hospital staff about them, but the inference leaves no room for doubt. However, God mercifully keeps us unaware of what lies ahead.

5

GOD'S FIRST RESPONSE

I was just reading in Hebrews this morning Lord. There is something about Hebrews that just kind of grates on me (no offense). It must have been written by some high powered preacher or one of those arrogant attorneys who think they are right about everything and then it turns out that they actually are! Quite irritating, but I have to admit that once I get past my prejudice, there are some parts that just knock my socks off if you know what I mean. Well of course you do. You're the one who wrote it. My only small complaint is that I wish you had given it to Paul to write. Now there's someone who is anything but an arrogant attorney type. Funny thing though, he started out that way; arrogant I mean, and just down-right mean at the same time. Amazing how a man can change like that! Not strange to you, I guess, especially since you made the whole thing happen. Happened just the way you wanted it too. Knocked Paul down several notches and then lifted him back up all the way to heaven at one point! Man! You certainly are God aren't you! Like I was saying though, I was reading in the eleventh chapter of Hebrews this morning and a couple of sentences just kicked me in the shins. Just to remind you here's what you said:

"All these people were still living by faith when they died. They did not receive the things promised; they only saw them and welcomed them from a distance."

I hate the sound of that! It means that I may not receive everything that I want in this life, including keeping my daughter Kelsey here with me. Do you really need her that badly up there? Are you sure there isn't someone else who could do her job for another 75 or 80 more years? I guess what you're telling me Lord is that faith is believing but also waiting for better things to come.

Crap!

I don't like that concept at all! It flies against my basic human nature. After all, didn't someone famous once tell us that we could have it all? I mean, she was talking to women about it, but I know she meant it for us men too. Why shouldn't I be able to get the things I want by investing my time, working hard, and praying like crazy? That seemed to work when I was building my career. Why doesn't it seem to be working for Kelsey? You know I've been praying hard, real hard. And lots of other people have been praying too. Surely you've heard us. Maybe we could talk louder. Maybe we only think we're praying hard. That's probably it. We just need to put more energy into our prayers.

Uh oh!

I'm getting the feeling that you're becoming a little impatient with me Lord. There's a little voice that's beginning to increase in volume. Now I'm beginning to sweat!

What was that?

In answer to your original question John, I don't mean to be wishy-washy, but yes and no. I have given you the capability to get the things that you want in your life on earth, but sometimes what you want is not what you need and believe it or not, to your good fortune I have to step in. Even when I know that giving you what you need is going to knock you to your knees. Believe me, it hurts me more than I can possibly have you understand when I feel that I must handle something this way. You know that every tear you've cried over Kelsey has fallen right into my hand. I haven't missed a single one and every one of your tears has brought a tear to my own eye. And since when did you start speaking for either God or Kelsey? How do you know what she and I have or haven't discussed during her illness? Why do you think you know more about what both you and Kelsey need than I do? Remember your place, and especially remember mine. I created Kelsey. I had a plan for her long before she ever came to you. Have you forgotten what you told me the night she was born? Don't you remember how happy you were that I did not take either Kelsey or Suzanne that night, even though they were both so close to coming home to me? Believe me, it could have gone either way that night. I listened to you then because it was what you needed at the time. You needed desperately for Kelsey and Suzanne to survive and stay with you. I made it happen. Once again though, I'm asking if you remember what you said to me that night? No? Well let me remind you. You said that I had given you a chance to see Kelsey and that if I decided to take her that night you would be okay with it. You do remember don't you? Well, what if I now decide it's time to take her fourteen years later? What has changed since then?

Lord, please forgive me, but a lot has changed. I don't want to be disrespectful, but I have had all these years to grow in my love for Kelsey. You let me continue to know her and watch her grow and love her more each year she has been with us. How horribly cruel to allow that and then snatch her away!

My point exactly John. I could have taken Kelsey that night; very few expected her to survive, and Suzanne had lost so much blood...well, I'm sure you remember. Remember also John, that my gift to you has been having the opportunity to love Kelsey for all these years. Would you have had me not give you that opportunity? You can't have it both ways and you don't always get what you want - not in this life anyway. You do remember my son don't you? Believe me, you did not have to stand by and watch Kelsey beaten to a bloody pulp, hung on a cross, ridiculed and spit on only to have her think, if only for a second, that you had abandoned her. Why do you think I did that John? Why do you think I was willing to sacrifice my one and only son that way? I think you know, but let me remind you anyway. I did it for one reason. I gave up my son to horrible abuse because I love you. End of story, bottom line. Let me repeat.

BECAUSE...I...LOVE...YOU.

Did you get that? Oh and by the way. Read the last part of that passage you began with John. You guys are always taking a piece of what I've said and leaving out the most important part. Notice that it says:

"And they were aliens and strangers on earth."

What?

Lord, you mean you created me and put me here on this planet, this earth, even though you knew I would be a stranger here? I thought you loved me and and wanted the best for me. I have been told Lord, and I truly believe that you are the creator of all things. Although I am beginning to wonder after all we have been through with Kelsey. So I ask you with respect, why put me where I apparently don't belong, in a place where terrible things will happen to me? And And once again Lord, I really hope you're OK with me asking these questions. I know it could be very dangerous for me if you're not!

John, I meant for you to be there. I meant for you all to be there, beginning with my first human creation. Oh how much I meant for Adam and Eve to be there from the very beginning! I prepared such a wonderful place for you all, with all of the things that you needed for a perfect and joyful life without the fear of death. I left nothing out, including the fruit for eternal life. I loved this place that I created so much that I would spend early evenings strolling the garden that I had given to Adam and Eve. Not only that, but I made mankind the overseer, the ruler of this kingdom. And John, there will be a day when I will once again stroll through the garden with those I love so dearly. With you John. There will be no more death. But that time is not here yet.

Only I know when these things will come to pass. But...

Well, here's what I instructed my good friend and obedient servant John to say after I scared him half to death on the isle of Patmos. He was there because of me you know. John and I have such wonderful times together now. He fought for me and stayed with me right up to the end. He's always been one of my favorites, right along with

Paul, Timothy, Peter, Rodger, Sam...Well, it's a long list. I am deeply in love with all of my children. In fact, you are all my favorites! but I digress... As I was saying, I instructed John to tell the following story. It is included in the book called Revelation. Quite an appropriate name don't you think? I did a really good job naming that one if I do say so myself. It is important enough that I want you to read it, contemplate it and write it on your heart. As always though, whether you do this or not is your choice. I always give you a choice. As I was saying, here's what I told John to write, and the beginning of an answer to your question. "And there was war in heaven. Michael and his angels fought against the dragon and the dragon and his angels fought back. But he was not strong enough and they lost their place in heaven. The great dragon was hurled down, that ancient serpent called the devil or Satan, who leads the whole world astray. He was hurled to the earth and his angels with him. Then I heard a voice in heaven say, Now have come the salvation, and the power, and the kingdom of God, and the authority of His Christ.*

For the accuser of our brothers, who accuses them before our God day and night, has been hurled down...Therefore, rejoice you heavens and you who dwell in them! But woe to the earth and the sea because the devil has gone down to you. He is filled with fury because he knows that his time is short...Then the dragon was enraged at the woman and went off to make war against her offspring - those who obey God's commandments and hold to the testimony of Jesus."

Do you see it? Does it make sense? It should, you know that I don't make mistakes.

6

DOWN THE RABBIT HOLE

There is a day, or more specifically an event in my memory that resides with several others of great emotional impact during the days of your illness. It is a reasonably warm fall afternoon and you and I are in the back yard enjoying the sun. It is the day after you have returned home from the hospital following a week long treatment. We both look at the rope swing in the tree and you look back at me and ask if I will push you in the swing. My answer of course is "sure." You are weak and your shoulder is still extremely sore from the biopsy. The infusion port is still sore as well. It has only been a short time since it was surgically implanted in your chest to allow for the frequent rounds of chemotherapy. As I lift you onto the swing, you look at me and state that even though you are weak, you feel pretty good today and want to take advantage of all the "good days" that you can. You and I are both painfully aware that the "good days" are becoming sparsely scattered in the sea of weeks in which you swim. Once you are seated and I have given you your first push, I turn momentarily to ensure that you will not see the tear that escapes and moves down my cheek. As I turn back to the swing, I am struck in a profound way, by the maturity in your statement. You are only nine! My forty five year old heart is breaking and my maturity is declining with each passing day. In contrast, as the treatments continue and the road becomes more difficult, your maturity and clarity about your condition seem only to solidify and grow. My heart breaks, and my faith and resolve falter just as your heart, resolve and faith continue to grow stronger. You seem to operate in a world that has no room for melancholy or self pity. In fact when asked why you think you got cancer, your answer is "So that my family could be an example for others." You responded to your school counselor that "The devil didn't realize what kind of little girl he was messing with when he made me sick!" What an inspiration you are and will continue to be in the days ahead.

The days ahead quickly become the days of now. It seems that you are in the hospital so much of the time Kelsey. It breaks my heart to see you pulled out of school and forced to spend the bulk of your time away from the friends that you love. The days seem to roll right into weeks which inevitably roll into months. Before we know it camp Esperanza time is here and you want desperately to go. We have been told by many doctors and nurses that this is a camp for kids with cancer, and that it is a wonderful experience because you will spend a week away from us and the hospital with a large group of other children who are experiencing much the same life as you. You will certainly not stand out at this camp as you feel you do everywhere else you go. There is one problem however you have been in the hospital all week with an infection that began when you became neutrapenic. Over the course of your treatment we have come to understand that neutrapenic means your white blood cell count is far too low leaving your body open to infection. This is a result of the poison you are receiving killing the good cells along with the cancer cells. You are still running some fever and the doctors will not let you go unless your fever subsides before tomorrow morning. You are heartbroken. You and the nurses have been talking about camp for days now and you are so excited about going. We are blessed however, and your fever is gone the following morning. It is extremely difficult for your mother as we load you on one of several buses to head down the highway for camp. She cries as you pull away, knowing in spite of the tears that this will be a great week for you. In fact, Camp Esperanza quickly becomes one of your favorite places, and camp week becomes something that you look forward to all year. Once you return from camp, the treatments seem to run together along with the countless infections, nausea, days without eating and many other side effects that come to define your life during this year of treatment. There are countless MRI's, breathing treatments and injections as well. The injections become my responsibility and they become as painful for me as they are for you. It is imperative that you receive them however, to stimulate your bone marrow to produce white blood cells. They must be given in your leg which makes them painful and unwanted. It breaks my heart to see the pain and tears that I feel responsible for as I force the needle into the sensitive skin of your thigh.

It continues to be a year filled with difficulties, lengthy hospital stays, and brutal treatments. You are unfortunately in the hospital more than you are out which results in your inability to attend school to any measurable degree. It is one more loss that inevitably extracts an emotional toll. You love being around your friends and this separation I know is difficult for you. It is just one more unforeseen consequence of your treatment protocol. We seem to have been so naïve about the implications and the context of your treatment. There are so many outcomes that we just could have never predicted. However, ignorance is indeed bliss in this case. Had we known the difficulties that faced us as we headed down this road together as a family, we may well have thrown in the towel early on. We stayed steady however, thanks in large part, to your remarkable resiliency and positive frame of mind throughout this year of frequent ups and downs. Following your worst periods of sickness, you invariably rebound to once again enjoy the good days that God has graciously given. During this year of treatment and the ensuing surgery to remove the tumor on your shoulder blade, there is always a light at the end of the tunnel. We are all working towards a powerful goal; the end of your treatment and the resulting death of your cancer. We all maintain a persistent optimism throughout your protocol based primarily on the belief that you can beat this thing. This optimism is most often the result of your own positive frame of mind, and the powerful impact that it has on each of us. Your mother spends hour after hour at the hospital with you whereas I come to see you in the evenings following work. There is a routine that we develop this year that becomes comforting in its own odd way. Powerful and supportive relationships with hospital staff members are developed, which brings an odd sense of security and hope.

The nurses in particular become valued and trusted friends. At last however, your treatment ends and following countless MRI's, hospital stays, injections, the indignities of poking and prodding every inch of your body, and emergency room visits, you are pronounced cancer free. What a wonderful time it is. I meet with your oncologist the day following your last treatment and he paints a realistic picture of what lies ahead. There will be many more MRI's for at least two years following your final treatment. The oncologist pulls me aside and informs me that he is optimistic about your cure, but he is also honest about the relatively strong chance for a recurrence. If the cancer should return, it will present us with a daunting challenge. Removing the disease a second time is considerably more difficult than the first. As the oncologist says, your chances for survival are markedly lower following a recurrence. This is not surprising information but it does put a damper on the day. I do not share this conversation with your mother until we have a few days of space between your release and your return to a life that will only resemble the one you left behind.

7

ANOTHER CONVERSATION

Lord I'm in pain. I have fallen into a seemingly bottomless pit. I have tried to climb out Lord, but I just keep falling back in, and each time I try it seems to get deeper and more difficult to claw my way up. Lord why must I suffer this way? What is the point? Better yet, what has Kelsey done to deserve this? We are good people Lord. We have done our best to live as you desire; To do good. What has Kelsey ever done but love you?

Are you finished yet John?

Yes. For now.

John, how do you know Kelsey's suffering? You know what you see, but you see little. Do you remember Habakkuk, John? Look again, and

notice my answer to his complaint. Better yet, do you even remember his complaint?

"Lord, how long must I ask for help and you ignore me? I cry out to you about violence, but you do not save us! Why do you force me to look at evil, and stare trouble in the face day after day? People are destroying things and hurting others in front of me. Anarchy and violence break out, quarrels and fights all over the place. Law and order fall to pieces. Justice is a joke. The wicked have the righteous hamstrung and stand justice on its head... God, why are you silent now? Holy God, You aren't going to let us die are you? This is outrage! Evil men swallow up the righteous and you stand around and watch!

God's Answer:

"Look! look around at the Godless nations. Look long and hard. Brace yourself for a shock. Something's about to take place and you're going to find it hard to believe... World conquering Babylon, grabbing up nations right and left. A dreadful and terrible people, making up its own rules as it goes... They descend like vultures circling in on Carion. They are out to kill. Death is on their minds...

Habakkuk wanted to know why I would allow an evil, violent and perverse nation to torture and murder him along with most of the Jewish people. John, Habakkuk was a righteous and honorable man. I was ready to allow him to suffer and die right along with the rest of his people. And you know what? I warned him before hand about his coming pain. Do you know how he responded to this? Well listen to Habakkuk in his own words, after he had an opportunity to calm down:

"Even if the fig tree does not bloom and the vines have no grapes, even if the olive tree fails to produce and the fields yield no food, even if the sheep pen is empty and the stalls have no cattle. Even then I will be happy with the Lord. I will truly find joy in God who saves me. The God of the Angel Armies is my strength. He makes my feet like those of a deer. He makes me walk on the mountains."

And now listen to Paul, John, and remember that he wrote this while chained to two guards. Paul had plenty of time to contemplate his trial and seemingly certain death:

"To me the only important thing about living is Christ, and dying would be even better for me. If I *continue to live in my body, I will be able to work for the Lord. I do not know what to choose - living or dying. It is hard to choose between the two..."*

John, don't project your feelings into my relationship with Kelsey, and don't confuse your feelings and desires with hers. I've mentioned this before, but unfortunately you're being a bit stubborn about understanding. Do you know how Paul died, John? Well, I guess that's an unfair question. The ones who knew have already left this earth, and it is not recorded in my word. Let's just say that Paul lost his mind so to speak. In other words, to be blunt, since that seems to be the only way to get through to you, Paul had his head unnaturally separated from his body.

Now do you think I don't love Paul?

I know you do Lord.

Then John, why would I let him die that way? And why would Paul say not long before he left his life on earth: *"My life is being given as an offering to God, and the time has come for me to leave this life. I have fought the good fight. I have finished the race. I have kept the faith. Now, a crown is being* *held for me - a crown for being right with God. The Lord, the judge who judges rightly, will give the crown to me on that day."*

You know, my son Jesus told many stories while He was taking care of my business on earth. Maybe a modern day story will help cement your understanding on this:

It was Mexico City 1968. John Steven Akhwari of Tanzania had started the Olympic marathon with all the other runners hours before, but he finished it alone. When he finally arrived at the stadium there were only a few spectators remaining in the stands. The winner of the marathon had crossed the finish line over an hour earlier. It was getting dark; his right leg was bandaged and heavily bleeding. He was obviously in great pain, but he crossed the finish line suffering from fatigue, leg cramps, dehydration, and disorientation. A reporter asked him why he didn't just quit. He thought for a moment and said, "My country did not send me here to start the race; my country sent me here to finish it."

John, I did not give Kelsey, Paul, Habakkuk or any of my other precious children the gift of life just to start the race. I created you to finish it.

Not only to finish it, but to finish strong, regardless of when your time to finish comes.

Paul finished strong. Kelsey finished strong. Habakkuk finished strong along with all the prophets and many others. They have and will receive great reward for that.

I understand Lord, but I am still struggling with why. Why did you make it this way? Why do we have to "endure" until we finish? Jesus Himself said "I came that they may have life and have it to the full." I know there is joy to be found, I just can't see the light at the end of the tunnel yet.

John, John, John! You are so fortunate that I am a God of compassion, patience and boundless love.

I will address that with you when we talk again...

8

A WELCOME RESPITE

Hey girlfriend,

How have you been doing since I last talked to you? What did you get for Christmas? I got a Papasoun Chair (it's the round one with wicker frame and the cushion that sits down in it).

Did you get what you wanted? I can't remember if I told you about this girl, named Courtney, that I met at the hospital, I don't think I did. She was on the same chemo I am, but it was not working for her. She had to stop and go on another one. Will you pray for her? She and I both would be very happy if you did. Thank you! The reason I told you about her was because she reminds me of you. I can only hope that she and I can have as good a friendship as we do. I miss seeing you, almost everyday, like we did when we were younger. I wish we could turn back time a couple of years to when we would go outside and ride bikes and play Barbie's. My favorite memories is sitting in the tree in my front yard and just talking. We'd sit there and talk for ever. I was thinking that you might be able to come out this summer. That would be sooooo cool! I was wondering if you had text messaging on your phone. If you do you can text me because I have unlimited. I would love to be able to talk to you

that way, and if you have e-mail
address or instant messaging? Well, talk
to you later.

Your friend forever,

Kelsey Wood

E-mail- shortie09_3@hotmail.com

Aol I.M.- shortie20093

Msn I.M.- shortie09_3

Following your first year of treatment, the
next days, months and ultimately two years are
filled with test, and many anxious times waiting for
the results of those test. Every test brings the
recollection of my conversation with your
oncologist following the end of your cancer
protocol. The anxiety flows from the knowledge
that any sign of cancer on one of these frequent
test, could mean the end of your life. The anxious
times however, are balanced by days of peace, days
of joy and days of thankfulness for a God who has
continued to cradle us in His arms during the worst
of times. As we all look back on your year of
treatment, we are amazed and at times bewildered

by the changes your illness has brought to our lives. Not that we are cynical, but we are not the family we spent so many years building and being. Even as we celebrate your freedom from treatment at a "Kelsey Kicks Chemo" party, we realize that there is an innocence that has been redefined as a cautious optimism. We are now quite familiar with the brutality that we have seen evident in the lives of others as they have traveled roads of difficulty visited upon them through an apparently random selection process; A cosmic role of the dice as it were. Or was it?

Thoughts of this nature are common as we move into this year of spiritual and emotional healing. As you move out of treatment I realize that you are only ten Kelsey, but you seem much older than that. You have lived half a lifetime in the past year as do most children who encounter this process. Growing up quickly is not an option but a necessity. I am so excited to be done with chemo, and all of the hospital time. We can now return to a semi-normal life. You are able to return to school to be with all of your friends. This is a wonderful thing in most respects, but you soon find that your friends have changed during your absence. It will be our first understanding that in many ways your life, as well as ours, will never again be the same. School will be difficult for you from this point forward. Socially, you must readjust to relationships that have moved forward without you. One relationship remains intact however, and that is the friendship that you share with your wonderful buddy Amanda. From our first week in the neighborhood, you and Amanda have gravitated to each other. Whether it is riding bikes, sharing secrets, or playing with Amanda's brothers and sisters, your days have been filled with the sweet friendship of youth. When you return home following treatment, you and Amanda seem to pick back up right where you left off. It is so wonderful to see you once again riding bikes, climbing trees, and hanging out with Amanda in the front yard sharing girl things that I know nothing about. Amanda will be your good friend and solid rock during the next two years. She was there for you when you were diagnosed and will remain with you until her family moves to Austin. Even following the move, you are able to visit her and she you. We will also make a major family move during this time when we decide to sell our home and build another in a more rural area.

During the year following treatment we will discover that for the first time you begin to struggle academically. Some of this we surmise, is due to the huge chunk of class time that you lost as a result of your treatment. Some struggles we will learn later, result from a learning disability that we were clueless about during your first years of school. Though I am now a principal, your mother and I will struggle with the fine line between supporting you with teachers and administrators and allowing you to struggle some on your own. During this time, we will come to know some wonderful teachers and administrators, as well as some who show no regard for you or your struggles with physical and academic disabilities. From the outside you look fine. Physically, your difficulties result from the inevitable chemotherapy recovery process which left you depleted and consistently tired. Your mobility is limited as well, as the result of the surgical removal of your scapula, and a reconstruction process that included severing and reattaching various muscles and ligaments. Because you do not have outwardly noticeable physical limitations, there are teachers who seem to delight in making you feel bad when you can't perform physically at the level of other students. But you try. Even with the limitations, you do your best to be like everyone else. This is your greatest concern and one that will haunt me as well. Following diagnosis and treatment, you will struggle with the desire to reclaim the life of normalcy that you left behind. You want so desperately to fit in but there are teachers who will force you into situations where you become the focus of attention. This hurts you deeply, and as result, we hurt for you. It instills within me the resolve to never become a calloused educator with little outward concern for the emotional welfare of my students. It is inconceivable to me how one could profess to be an educator and yet show little concern for the emotional and spiritual well being of the students entrusted to his or her care.

For the better part of two years we are granted a blessed relief from the cruelty of your year-long protocol. Each visit to the clinic for scans brings anxious moments, and long waits for you and your mother as well as time away from school, but the news is good. Each visit finds no sign of the return of this vicious disease, and after each visit, we thank God for his favorable providence. We almost forget the harsh reality of the previous year. Almost, but not quite... In July of your second post treatment year, we sell our home across the street from Amanda, and move to a temporary address while construction on our new home is completed. It is a very small unit in a four-plex, and we are terribly cramped for space. Your brother sleeps in the den while you and your sister sleep in the second bedroom. It is far less than ideal, but you love it. You love it because we are forced into closeness as a family that brings your now high school age brother and sister great distress, but brings you great joy. You thrive on this closeness and will mention this time together often as one that you view with affection. July becomes August and much to our amazement, we wake up one morning to discover that we are firmly planted in the middle of October. October 2002. Two years from the end of your treatment and three years from your diagnosis in November of 1999. I don't know what it is about fall, but this one will once again rock our world.

9

WHERE IS GOD?

Prostate cancer is a strange beast. It took your grandfather Kelsey, but he might have dodged that bullet had he paid a bit more attention to his body and to your grandmother's advice. But it was not to be. He followed the path that was laid before him with grace and courage as did your grandmother. His last days were difficult, having become a shadow of what he once was, and frequently sinking into morphine induced alternate realities which eventually became his only reality. We could only imagine the life he was living behind the veil of morphine and pain. A pain that became so intense and unrelenting that he began to suffer in every reality. The morphine was no longer adequate to relieve the pain, leaving him dazed, confused, and wrapped in the grip of an unrelenting monster. His life eventually became a symphony of moans and cries as we attempted in every way possible to lessen his misery. As your grandfather's final days approached, I was forced to choose between several treatment options, all aimed at eliminating my cancer before I was forced to walk my father's pathway. At times it seemed the choices were limitless and confusing, but also encouraging.

When I entered our tiny apartment that November evening, I was a man with a treatable cancer and multiple treatment options. Your cancer was gone, and though my father was dying, we were coming to terms with his approaching death and planning for the future. Our prayers were being answered and God was at work in a positive way in the life of our family. Had He not showered us with two years of cancer freedom as evidenced by your frequent and disease free testing? We were cautious but very optimistic about your cure. Your two year cancer-free mark was a remarkably important signpost towards that goal. For two years, you had worked towards putting your life back together. School was difficult, but you had new friends as well as old. We were all resigned to the fact that cancer had irrevocably changed our lives into something entirely different, but increasingly positive. Positive however, resists definition and as we have previously experienced, life can change in the blink of an eye.

I am lying on the bed in our small apartment in the fetal position. The door is closed. I do not want either you or your brother and sister to see me this way Kelsey. I am hurting and trying to comprehend what I have just been told. I am praying. I am processing. I am trying to pull it all together before I return to the den. It's not working. Right now, all I want to do is lie here curled up, and bury myself in the enormity of our situation. I can't allow myself that luxury. You need me right now Kelsey as much as you have ever needed me. The rest of our family needs me as well. Your mother is there with you as always, providing what is to me, an unfathomable determination and calm support as we learn of this new development. Somehow after I have wallowed in my shock and hurt for a few minutes, God begins to plant seeds of hope. My resolve returns and begins to strengthen. I force my fears and hurts back and leave them alone in the bedroom. They will be there when I return, and in fact will follow me for the foreseeable future. Right now however, I still have the strength and the wherewithal to walk away. At some point I will continue talking to God about this and leave the fears and hurts with Him. Right now however, I have determined to rely on a temporary fix, and God patches me up and waits for my return for more extensive healing. I am clueless at this point, that the healing will be years down the road. As I begin to plan our next steps as a family, I am drawn to recall the events that forced us to the edge of this precipice upon which we now tenuously rest.

This current nightmare began the last week of October 2002 with your mother's surgery. It was not life threatening, but more extensive than her doctor originally anticipated. In keeping with your mother's typical stubbornness, and determination, she returned to work before the doctor released her, but never missed a beat once she was back on track. During her recovery, your grandfather's skirmish with prostate cancer became a full scale campaign with the cancer quickly driving him into surrender. His once slow and steady decline became a physical freefall leaving him in constant pain with a growing inability to eat. I could see the resignation inch its way into his once stubborn and confident resolve to beat this intrusion into his once unshakable life. He had given it his best shot, and could do no more. It was both heart breaking and comforting to see my beleaguered mother serve his needs daily as he progressed towards an unfavorable resolution to this unexpected intrusion into our lives. We just never thought of your grandfather as anything but able to beat the odds. As your uncles, your aunt and I all grew together from childhood to maturity, he became the rock that we assumed would never crumble, with your grandmother providing the behind the scenes support that would allow him to maintain that stability. Yes it was bad. But he had used his determination and positive outlook to beat back other challenges to his health and stability. We all thought this struggle would be no different. As his illness rapidly progressed, God began to use his deteriorating condition to precipitate a life saving work in my own life.

This work began innocently enough one evening as I perused books in the local library. As luck (read God) would have it, I stumbled upon a book on men's health by Dr. Kenneth Cooper, the well respected "father of aerobics." As I lay in bed one night thumbing through the pages, I began to read a chapter devoted to prostate issues and the accompanying symptoms of disease. It was a natural action based upon my father's ultimately fatal encounter with prostate cancer. As I read more deeply into the chapter, I became increasingly convinced that my own body had been invaded by this rotten disease that was about to claim my father. This realization manifested itself in spite of the complete lack of evidence to support the conviction. It was simply a matter of knowing that I had cancer. Nothing more, nothing less; I just knew (read God). Upon this realization I rolled over and scooted closer to your mother in bed. Much to her surprise, I proceeded to share my revelation and self diagnosis with her. Much to her credit, she did not dismiss my conviction and true to her nature, proceeded to reassure me, and suggest that I have a blood test done as the first step towards diagnosis. I took her advice Kelsey, as you most surely knew I would, and had the blood test done within the week. The results were back to me the following week. No major issues the urologist said. My PSA was up slightly but still well within acceptable limits. The reading indicated that there was a very small likelihood that cancer had invaded my body. In spite of the urologist's calm demeanor and equally reassuring words, a still, small voice began to speak to me. I told the urologist that in the face of evidence to suggest otherwise, I felt a biopsy was appropriate. He disagreed. I persisted and we scheduled a biopsy. For my own peace of mind the urologist said. He continued to feel certain that the biopsy was a formality and would reveal no cancer. I continued to believe that it would (read God). Approximately one week later, we both discovered that he was wrong. The phone in my office rang and I answered.

"Mr. Wood?"

"Yes."

"This is Doctor ...." I have good news and I have bad news. Which would you like first?"

My immediate thought was how about no news, but the words I heard myself speak were: "let's do the bad news first."

"The bad news is you have cancer. This was no shock to me, but obviously had taken the doctor by surprise.

"Doctor, what's the good news?"

"The good news is that the cancer is very small and confined to one lobe of your prostate gland. Let's make an appointment so I can further explain and we can discuss your options."

I felt blessed Kelsey. This was actually good news. It was a blessing that your cancer was gone and mine was small and treatable.

My dad's situation was not so favorable, but we would weather that storm and move forward as a family. I found new hope and new encouragement. In spite of my cancer, I was beginning to see a light at the end of the tunnel. Things were looking up...

I blinked this evening and experienced life screaming like a freight train; barreling through our

tiny apartment with the whistle at full blast,
demolishing everything in its pathway except us.
Instead, it leaves us broken, battered, and barely
alive with nothing of any substance to hold onto.
The foundation is gone and our lives lie in scattered
pieces all around us. Indeed, it feels as if we
have barely escaped with our lives and shortly your
mother and I will wonder if this life we are given is
a blessing or a curse. How do we move forward and
live from here? Will we even be able to refer to the
lives we now face as truly living or just existing?
The questions come quickly and without mercy,
pelting us like hail as it rains down from the sky.
Each question stings in a way that makes us wish
that it were actually physical pellets bombarding us
from above. We are up late.

Your mother sits and holds you. It is an image that
stands fixed in my imagination, and will take place
many times as we lurch forward into the coming
weeks. Watching you sit in your mother's arms is
comforting, yet disturbing. Disturbing because it is
always the result of bad news, of pain, of dejection,
of the futility of the battle that we are fighting. Is it
even a battle, or is that the best analogy that we

can construct to explain the bewildering and oppressive events taking place?

God only knows.

And tonight, for a brief time, I am not at all happy with His seeming lack of concern for you and for our family.

Where is He?

Where is God? is a recurrent theme, even though I push the thought out of my consciousness and back into the place where thoughts go to reside until they resurrect themselves at the worst possible time. At this point, I have not yet learned that difficult thoughts don't ever disappear, nor can we keep them hidden for the long term. They always rise back up out of the thought graveyard to wreak havoc on our weakened psyches until we confront them, wrestle with them, and ultimately come to terms with them. As I rise from the bed, however, I have been successful at replacing those thoughts with thoughts of strength and resolve. The news that put me here in this tiny bedroom lying curled up on the bed is devastating. Your cancer is back and has metastasized to your lungs.

MRI's don't lie, and your most recent one spoke loudly and clearly to this effect. Just minutes earlier, your mother's voice began to become distant and reverberate as she shared this news. As you leave to retreat to your room, I keep repeating the question, "Is there hope, did the oncologist say there was hope? It is an unfair question for your mother, and she informs me that the doctor will call that evening with more specific information and options. As bad as the news is, I am convicted that we will beat this beast. With God's divine intervention, as hopeless as it now seems, I believe with all my heart, that the cancer will disappear. It must. There is no other option.

10

THE LONG CLIMB UP

Lord, as each step hits the pavement and my legs begin to burn, I see the hill ahead and begin to mentally prepare for the long climb up. My legs already ache, and I seem unable to pull enough oxygen into my lungs to compensate for the outgo of carbon dioxide. I begin to tighten my muscles, and increase the frequency of my breaths in anticipation (or is it fear) of the hill ahead. As I hit the base, I look up only to realize that the ascent seems to summit at least a half mile ahead. How can I do this for half a mile? I'm already tired, I am only halfway into my run and now I'm confronted with a half mile climb that to my estimation becomes steeper towards the summit.

I can't do it.

I'll just quit.

That's it.

I will stop and walk up each of the hills, and only run on the downhills and flats. It's a good thought, but quickly disappears as I consider the consequences of "cheating" my way through the run. My teeth grind as I make my way up and begin to feel the pain involved in what now seems to be a foolhardy and doomed attempt to defeat this obstacle. Halfway up the hill my legs begin to burn unmercifully as I simultaneously realize that there is absolutely no way that I can suck enough air into my lungs to satisfy my oxygen starved body. My thought then jumps to the fact that even though I may make it to the crest of this hill without stopping, I will have depleted every physical resource that I have, leaving me decimated and unable finish my run. This pain is inescapable. There is no way around it, over it or under it. If I want to finish this six mile run, and I desperately do, the pain must be dealt with.

Then suddenly it makes sense.

Right smack in the middle of the hill, on the way to the ultimate crescendo of pain, it hits me full in the face. Relax, lean into the hill, breathe deep, and confront the pain. Better yet, don't stop to avoid the pain; don't run to the flat to escape the pain, run into the pain. It seems completely counterintuitive, but absolutely the right thing to do.

So I do it.

I begin to focus on the relaxation, breathing, and leaning into the hill. At some point, I lose track of these things and focus on the joy and the beauty of this run. I begin to contemplate the God- given physical blessings that allow me to experience this type of activity. Before I realize it, the pain does not disappear, but somehow becomes a clarifying lens through which I view the ultimate goal. The pain evolves into a sweet and defining test of my endurance. The goal then, becomes a combined effort of squeezing the painful joy out of a difficult climb and enduring to experience the sweet-spot of victory at the end. What an ah ha! experience. How can this be? How can difficulty and pain bring about anything uplifting and good? How can joy and pain be connected in any way, much less having joy derived from pain? I don't have the answers, but I do know that it is true. I experienced it on this run and look forward to the next painful, joy producing run. However, I now realize that it is not necessary to obtain a complete understanding of the process in order to benefit from the experience. This, I have come to realize, is the nature of trust. This is the beauty in God's statement to Paul:

"My strength comes into to its own in your weakness."

That's it! That's what you're telling me Lord, isn't it? When the hill seems insurmountable; when the pain is intense, and I am too weak to continue the climb, I am comforted and even joyful, as your strength lifts me up and over the hill.

What a load of crap!

What planet was I on during that run yesterday?

Lord, you know what I said about joy coming from pain yesterday? Well today it just feels like hell. I am digging deep for the joy but I can't see the top of the hill and the wind is blowing hard in my face. God, what do I have left? It just all seems to be falling apart, and I can barely see the light. How in the world does a person deal with such crushing, soul jarring, mind numbing events? I look at my sweet Kelsey, father and my heart aches in a physical way within my chest.

But wait...

Kelsey, is that really you? Are you really, truly standing in front of me smiling? Didn't you hear the news?

Don't you know that your chances for survival just diminished by seventy percent?

What in the world do you have to smile about? You must be absolutely crushed, defeated and miserable. You must be...

What?

You're telling me it's going to be ok? How do you know sweet baby?

A voice said what?

You were in the garage?

A voice spoke to you in the garage?

Surely this voice must have spoken words of greater wisdom from a place much more pleasant than a crowded garage with a dirty floor. That is if you actually did hear this voice saying those words. It must have spoken something more than "Kelsey, it will be ok."

No, you say?

You're telling me that's all you need to hear? You're satisfied, encouraged, and at peace with that?

You are truly incredible sweet child. Come here and sit next to me for a while. Yes, I believe that you did hear a voice, and whether it was God or an angel doesn't matter. You are not frightened, or upset. You are just incredibly sensitive to the voice of the one who gave you life; the one who may now stand by and watch while your life is taken away.

I remember.

Yes, it is crystal clear now. The day three years ago in the backyard, when you asked me to push you in the tire swing because you were having a good day and you wanted to squeeze every last drop of joy out of that day that God would allow. Though there was pain, and sickness, there was also joy.

Incredible. Truly incredible.

How do you do it Kelsey? How do you squeeze out that joy in the midst of the pain? I thought I knew, but I don't. I feel depressed and defeated. Here you are however, speaking of an encouraging voice and simply, passionately enjoying the moment. There are tears in my eyes, and heaviness in my heart.

God, please say it won't end.

Please tell me that I will have many more years to sit with this sweet child and talk of things that we will both treasure in our hearts.

You can't do this God! You can't take her away.

Please let her stay.

I am pleading Lord. Can't you hear me?

Where are you God?

11

SLIDING BACK DOWN

I know where God is. He's with you, Kelsey. His Spirit and His kingdom are very much at work within you. As we move into this next phase of treatment, your mother and I huddle together to plan and to gain strength from each other. We approach the coming days with solid resolve and determination to continue our forward progress on a day by day basis in thought and action. The scan shows only three very small spots on one of your lungs. Your oncologist tells us there is no way to know the certainty of this information without invading your chest to take a look. He tells us the surgery will be difficult and the recovery long and arduous. He talks to you first as he always does and bluntly but compassionately, provides you with information and options. He then turns to your mother and I, and speaks to the three of us in summary. When he leaves the room to let us discuss the information he has just shared with us, we decide to move forward with the lung biopsy, and a date is set. The surgery is successful, but extremely difficult, and the recovery is every bit as difficult as anticipated. This will be the first of two lung surgeries that coupled with the radiation, will leave you with permanent lung damage. In retrospect, your mother reflects that given another opportunity, she would not have voted for the second surgery. However, that decision would have been based on a great deal of additional information that was unavailable at the time. After discussion with the clinical team, we are able to convince them to allow your new chemotherapy protocol to be done at home. As a result, we all become quite proficient with pieces of the process that had previously been done by a medical professional. The hospital staff continued to insert the large needle into the port that had been surgically placed in your chest, but your mother and I became co-conspirators in the painful removal of the needle following each round of chemotherapy. We continue to maintain hope and optimism for your recovery. This protocol proceeds for six months during which I have prostate cancer surgery and you receive a round of radiation to provide a more powerful attack on the tumors.

This six month protocol begins a two year roller coaster ride of clinical trials, treatment protocols, hopes and dreams, as well as nightmares, fear, and fractured hope. There were so many scans, hospital stays, and unique and varied treatments during this period of time, that your mother and I can no longer recall specific times and dates for them all. You encountered each of them with courage, hope and an unwavering faith in God's sovereignty and grace. Your words were always positive and reflective of a bright future. However, to your beloved aunt Karen, you intimated that you were quite sure that you did not want to continue with this disease into young adulthood. You also did research on brain tumors, which we considered at the time to be completely out of the realm of possibility for your type of cancer. Statistically, the odds that Ewing's sarcoma would metastasize to the brain were infinitesimally small.

There are certainly events during this period of time that characterize themselves as important and impactful, and still resound with clarity in our thoughts and hearts. Many wonderful prayers were offered in your behalf, and many wonderful and caring people continued to visit you during the frequent hospital stays. One of the experimental treatments that you received on an outpatient basis, allowed us all to meet a wonderful young man named John, who was receiving treatment in the same infusion room, at times just a chair or two away from yours. John was twenty and was receiving

treatment as a last resort in his struggle with
Ewing's sarcoma. Whether as a form of spiritual
and psychological self defense, or self protection
through denial, we did not completely
understand at the time that you were receiving
this treatment as a "last ditch effort" as well. This
is where the memories become very fuzzy, and
manifest themselves in fragments lodged like
random bricks in the structure of our psyches,
but somehow disconnected from the whole. Your
mother and I lost contact at some point with the
exact sequence of events and treatment. One
random event however that stays with us to this
day Kelsey is the conversation we had with the
nurse in charge of your medical trial protocols. I
am certain that she is a decent person, but her
callousness was sometimes disconcerting. At one
point she intimated to the three of us that given
the diagnosis of an aggressive cancer, she would
prefer to simply die rather than endure the
habitual and debilitating effects of treatment. At
another time, she verbally reflected on the futility
of John's treatment since he would surely "die
anyway." You were present for both of these

comments and to your credit, took each in stride, with no comment regarding either. The scans during each of the treatments were ever changing and deceptively encouraging at times. We would anxiously anticipate the report from each and cheer for each scan that reflected evidence of tumor stability or reduction. Your oncologist was gentle, compassionate and judicious as he gently led us to the ultimate conclusion regarding your condition. As gentle as he was however, I refused to believe his prognosis, and trusted God to provide for your healing regardless of the severity and hopelessness of your condition. God is good, and you are a wonderful, spiritual, believing young lady. He has heard our prayers, and there is no question in my mind, that He will respond to those prayers in a powerful and positive way, in spite of the doctor's prognosis to the contrary. If I believe intensely and unswervingly, He will provide us with

our desires, and what we desire is for you to be free of this vile disease.

12

YOU'RE NOT COMING HOME

To all of her friends and prayer warriors out there, Kelsey Wood sends her greetings. She wanted me to tell all of you how much she loves you, and to not worry about her. She's dancing with Jesus today.

Paul says in II Corinthians 12, *"I know a man, in Christ who fourteen years ago was caught up to the third heaven. Whether it was in the body or out of the body I don't know, but God knows. And*

I know that this man-whether in the body or apart from the body I don't know, but God knows-was caught up to paradise. He heard inexpressible things, things that man is not permitted to tell."

Sometime on Wednesday evening March 2, 2005, amidst the clamor and beeps of the Children's Medical Center emergency room, it is my belief that Kelsey Wood experienced some form of what Paul is describing here. My faith is not diminished by the fact that as much as she knew we wanted to have her back, Kelsey and God decided that it was best for her not to return to this world. Even as Kelsey took her last breath, I believed and continue to believe, that God could override all of the physical issues involved and bring her back. I believe that he has done this in our day and time. I believe as well, that what she experienced was so beautiful, and her faith in us to continue in strength without her so strong, that she understandably did not want to come back.

I want to thank all of you who stood firm in prayer. To all of those who stood in the gap for

Kelsey by praying in faith for her with firm belief in God's power to heal, please understand that your prayers were not ignored.

Once again, my faith in God and his ability to override any earthly roadblocks and provide total and complete healing in any situation remains unchanged. I will continue to pray in the spirit for God's intervention in seemingly impossible situations.

"For it is God who works in you to will and to act according to his good purpose." **Philippians 2:13**

God has worked and is continuing to work through Kelsey to achieve His good purpose.

In Christ,

John Wood

Spoken to the assembly at Rolling Hills Church of Christ Sunday morning March 6, 2005

13

DARKNESS DESCENDS

The call came late in the afternoon. It was obvious from the tone of your mother's voice that something was terribly wrong.

"Kelsey's in trouble, I'm on my way to the hospital." On the way out the door she breathlessly explained that you had been changing the curtains in your bedroom, when you noticed a tingling in your right arm and leg.

You limped into the den and asked "Mom am I too young to have a stroke?" You then told her that your right arm and leg were, "feeling really weird." In the following seconds they continued to become numb and useless. I immediately moved from my office to the front desk to let the school know that I was rushing out to meet you and your mother at the hospital.

As the miles and minutes clicked by, I remember praying fervently for God to let you survive this. Over and over I prayed the same desperate prayer, "Please God, let this not be serious, let Kelsey survive this." I could think of nothing else to pray. I pulled into the emergency room parking area, jumped from my car, and ran for the emergency room door. As I passed through the door in a panic, I began to search for you and your mother. As I moved through the hallway, I saw your mother at the front desk and ran to her side. As I listened it became clear that she was attempting to obtain a wheel chair to get you inside. She turned and asked me to go to the parking lot and check on you. I ran back out the emergency room door and found you in the passenger seat. As I opened the door to the car, I immediately began to reach for you and ask how you were. In the intensity of that moment, I quickly realized that you could not, and would not respond to my words. Nothing could have prepared me for the impact of the sight before me. As I reached for you and looked in your eyes, I noticed that your pupils were three to four times their normal size, at the same time the sight and smell of vomit assaulted my senses. The front of your wind suit was covered in it. My heart literally shattered in that moment, as my soul cried out at the injustice and the frightening and pitiful nature of your condition. I will never in this life, forget that moment in time, as I once again silently screamed out at God for my complete and utter inability to mediate your horrifying condition. To helplessly watch one of your children suffer in a way that you could never have imagined is a soul shattering, heart breaking experience. The picture of that moment has become a nightmare that won't disappear. Unlike a photo, it can never be destroyed or deleted.

Following a great deal of effort, we are able to obtain a wheelchair and roll you into the emergency room ourselves. It amazes me how little help we are given by the emergency room staff. They ignore most of our pleas that you are dying and should be placed in a treatment room. As you sit in the waiting room, unable to communicate and slowly slipping away from us, I give up on the emergency room staff and make a run for the elevator to possibly find a staff member on the sixth floor cancer unit. Incredibly, I run into one of the oncologists who just happens to be the only staff member left on the floor and one who is familiar with you and your case. I breathlessly relate your situation to her, and her calm but chilling response of "that's very troublesome" does not encourage me. Once on the emergency room floor, she quickly gets you into a treatment room, and pulls several other staff members in with her. They hook you up and begin to monitor your vital signs as your mother and I observe. You are well past the ability to speak, but as the oncologist ask you if you know where you are and what is happening you

respond by moving your head in a signal for yes.
The oncologist who began this journey with us
and has continued to be your kind and caring
medical partner throughout this devastating five
and one half year struggle, has been notified and
arrives in your treatment room. He walks to your
bedside, asks a few questions, looks at the
reports, and gently takes your hand. As he looks
into your eyes and checks for recognition, he asks
if you understand how serious your condition is.
You respond by once again moving your head to
signify yes. He then tells you that you are in grave
condition and the outcome quite probably will
not be what any of us want.

The oncologist who rushed to your side from
the cancer floor, looks in my direction and
indicates for me to meet her in the hospital
hallway. As I move out of the room, somehow I
unknowingly position myself with my back to the
wall. The oncologist then moves to face me and
rests both of her hands on my shoulders. As I
stand looking into her eyes, she calmly states that
I should understand that you may not survive the
night. Having never fainted, I was unprepared for

my response to this news. Fortunately my back was against the wall as my world faded to black and I collapsed to the floor. It is impossible to describe the profound and devastating impact of the realization that your child is near death. Three days later as I watched you inhale and not release the breath, I knew that you were gone, but in my heart I believed that God could still raise you up off that bed if he chose to. All those days and nights of prayer; surely God was not going to be complicate in your death. Surely the prayers had meant something to him and he would not allow you to be taken from us. It was not to be. Your last breath came the day following our decision to bring you home under hospice. It was as if you were telling us "No offense guys, but I really don't want to do it that way. I'm ready to move on and God is ready to have me. I don't want any delays." That would be just like you Kelsey. You never delayed in decisions and you were obviously ready to meet the one who was not only your God, but your trusted friend. In retrospect, I believe that you saw God, or maybe his representatives before you took that last breath. I could see it on your face and by the look in your eyes. Besides, when we visited the funeral home to make sure they had dressed and prepared you well for visitation, we complimented them for leaving you with the prettiest and most contented smile on your face. In fact, it was almost a smirk. The response from the funeral home director however, was that they had not done anything of the sort. He assured us that you had come to them with the smile already in place. I believe it appeared as a smirk when you actually saw the beauty before you and thought "Wow, you guys don't have a clue, but I do, and I'm on my way!"

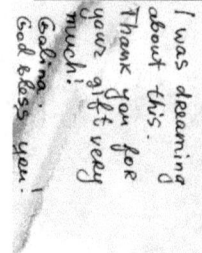

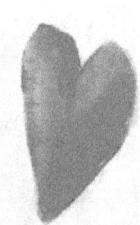

In the left margin (handwritten, vertical):
I was dreaming about this. Thank you for your gift very much! Galina. God bless you.

July 2005

In memory of KELSEY WOOD

From the young people at the church in Tallinn, Estonia,
which meets on Asunduse Street ...

We all wish to thank those of you who gave the CD player and Christian CDs
for us to enjoy.

Our hearts are touched with your grief because you had to bid a temporary
'good bye' to Kelsey as she returned to our Heavenly Father. We are
strengthened in faith as we share the hope and assurance of eternal life
with you. You will see Kelsey again, and we will meet her. Until then, with
eyes of faith we see her in the presence of God the Father and His
wonderful Son who loves children so very much. And, with ears of faith, we
hear her voice singing with angels.

We will listen to our songs of praise on our new CD player, remembering the
Wood family and Kelsey with love and thanksgiving.

Your brothers and sisters in Tallinn,

(In the right margin, handwritten vertically: Thank you! Stanley :)

Handwritten signatures:
Thank you so much! Hilli. Anna. Peter Jakai. Ron + Judy Warpole - with our love!
God bless you? God. Vadim Yakovlev - with our God.
Thank you! Sasha. Thanx!!! Julia =) Thank you! TY miss Kate (or simply #.)
Thank you very much! Anja
Thanks!!! guys... With love, Sandra. Liza. Thank you! Olga. Thanks a lot Katja =) Tsvetu c
Thank you Helen. Пламена Петрова. T.Belkina. Dan. Olga. We love you, God bless you. Stas I'm with you all!
Thanx! from Sveta and Andrej. Lilia. Thank you very much, We love u Oleg & Jelena

14

TIMING IS EVERYTHING

At the core of life and death is the battle
against our spirits. Satan, or his representative, is
always waiting and watching for an opportunity, any
small opening, to latch his bony claws around our
hearts and scratch and squeeze until we are literally
drained of blood and spirit. At this point, with every

ounce of strength and resolve drained, we figuratively (and at times literally), crumble into a heap on the ground. These are times when hope ruins scarce, and no matter what we try, nothing will bring us to a place of rest and peace.

We cannot shrink from these times.

Satan brings hell to earth and entices us to roll over and give in. He intensifies the attack by working on our thoughts; by taking old hurts and pains and magnifying them until we are literally bleeding emotionally and spiritually. By picking, poking and prodding with hurtful thoughts that begin small, but ultimately rise to a crescendo of pain.

"You may as well give up."

"You'll never be able to overcome this."

"You'll never be good enough."

"Things will never be the same."

"He will never love me again."

"What you had is gone forever."

"How could she cheat on me this way?"

"I'll never find another job."

Don't tell me that at some point, you haven't heard some of these voices. They are at times a roaring noise in our heads and at other times almost imperceptible, but still there. The problem is that sometimes the Spirit is a still, small voice, and Satan's blaring message can easily drown it out if we don't listen carefully. Listening is an essential component in the communication process, but in order to hear the voice we must first communicate our needs, then wait and listen. Waiting is difficult, especially when the pain is intense. It is nearly impossible; nearly, but not quite. We may think that we are unable to bear the pain, particularly when the negative thoughts flow almost imperceptibly from one into the other leaving us battered, bruised, and swimming in a sea of negativity. There is little room for a positive thought to squeeze itself into the tiny gap and the micro-second of time between the biting, hurtful lies perpetrated by the father of lies.

So what are we to make of this? What are we to understand about the spiritually, mentally, emotionally and physically devastating impact of catastrophic loss? What are we to make of the seemingly unrelenting assault on our thoughts and our spirits following catastrophic loss? First we should define catastrophic loss. Since no dictionary definitions exist to my knowledge, I am forced to rely on subjectivity based on personal experience, as well as the experience of others. For our purposes, let's define catastrophic loss as the removal of any key component in the context of our lives for any reason. The context can include death, divorce, loss of mobility (through paralysis), as well as any other number of losses that can precipitate unalterable and dramatic changes in our lives. Let's further define the loss as permanent. A loss which will leave a permanent emptiness that will never be filled. Other components may be added to our lives following the loss, but as excellent as these additions may be, the hole remains, and our lives may become wonderful and possibly even better in some ways than before, but never the same.

Is it even possible to find meaning in the loss? Were we singled out in some way for a specific reason, or can we just attribute the loss to some cosmic "roll of the dice" where you and I "crap out" so to speak? Though I know intellectually that God is sovereign, I am not at all comfortable with a God who at times acts in ways, or allows events to occur that are devastating to His children. I cannot deny that the universe and everything in it is His creation and He acts in the perfection of His own understanding and not ours. That intellectual understanding however, does nothing to soften the harshness of the loss, to ease my pain, or strengthen my faith. Those who say they are not angry at God for allowing such a catastrophic loss have not yet dug deeply into the core of the hurt, the anger and the resentment. Yes, at some point in the grieving process, we are angry at God, whether we choose to admit this fact or not. God let us down. He said that He would take care of us and answer our prayers. But He didn't. I prayed extensively and diligently and it apparently had no effect on God because He did not reach out in compassion and stop my loss. He did not heal Kelsey, and in fact, allowed her to suffer and die well before her time.

So what now?

Faith is much more than just believing that God will always respond to our prayers by giving us what we ask for. It is believing that God will do what is right even when we do not understand or agree. Is it fair? Absolutely not! Not fair but perfect. Faith **is** being certain that what God has promised is true. It is believing in the invisible.

Why believe His promises? Why trust in the invisible?

Why not?

It takes a tremendous "leap of faith" to believe in the insane notion that the universe somehow morphed into existence as the result of a chain of infinitely unlikely and random events.

To believe that the universe was spontaneously generated from an infinite void where no matter previously existed. It takes less faith to believe that something or someone had to exist before time, distance and matter and that this someone sparked the existence of time, distance and matter as we know it. "*Because of our faith, we know that the world was made at God's command. We also know that what can be seen was made out of what cannot be seen.*" Hebrews 11:3.

But believing is not enough. It's never enough. Particularly when our world begins to crumble and Satan whispers in our ear that God doesn't care. God makes no mistakes. My daughter Kelsey's death was not a mistake. It was not a matter of God looking back and saying, *oops, I can't believe I missed that prayer and let her die. I just waited too long to answer."*

Why did He wait to answer until after Kelsey had passed from this life, or until your husband left you for another woman or until the bankruptcy was final? Why did He wait to answer until cancer took your husband or wife?

Why, why, why...?

15

LET THE HEALING BEGIN

*Isaiah 57:1-2 'Those who are right with God
may die, but no one pays attention. Good
people are taken away, but no one understands.*

*Those who do right are being taken away from
evil and are given peace. Those who live as
God wants find rest in death."*

I woke following a dream last night; or early
this morning. I'm not sure because I did not look at
the clock. It was a simple dream, but one that I was
somewhat surprised to have. In my dream, I was

lying on my bed in conversation with my wife Suzanne who was in another area of our bedroom. At some point in the dream, I began to sob and cry out "It still hurts so badly after four years. Why does it still hurt so much after so much time?" Suzanne did not respond and I continued to sob and cry out the question several more times. No talking animals or strange and unusual imaginary creatures or events. Instead, there was just a painful realization that in spite of the passage of time, I still continue to puzzle over the answers to these simple questions. Even this morning, I continue to recall the pain of the dream quite clearly. There are places, occasions, smells, songs, and other sensory triggers that send an immediate dagger piercing into the soft spots of the memories and grief that still remain. This is as it should be. However, I do not think about Kelsey all the time, and in fact there are days that I do not think of her at all. This is as it should be. She would want nothing less. My wife Suzanne and I do not have daily conversations about Kelsey either with each other or with friends and family. This is as it should be. Once again, Kelsey would want nothing less. I surmise that over the passage of time, I have attempted to relegate at least some thoughts of Kelsey and the questions that I continue to ponder regarding her death, to a bookshelf of previously read material. I have completed the books but still do not have complete understanding of their contents. I have thus shelved them in my subconscious where I do not have to deal with them consistently or consciously. At times apparently, in the unguarded and emotionally exposed world of dreams, they rise again to force my consideration.

I am never quite sure whether this is nefarious or divine, and I suppose that it is not particularly relevant either way. Of particular relevance however, is how I choose to deal with these dreams and their potential impact on my waking life. I choose to consider them briefly and to move forward. One dream in particular blurred the line between divine and demonic. I still recall it quite clearly which may indicate that it will reappear at some point to revisit me again. Once again, it was a simple yet emotionally powerful dream. Out of deference for my wife Suzanne, and the possible emotional fallout that the dream might engender in her, I have chosen not to share it until now. In my dream, I was sitting in a car with Kelsey, who appeared somewhat younger than the fourteen years that she had accumulated at the time of her death. At some point in the dream, our innocuous and positive ride was punctuated by Kelsey's clearly painful cry, *"I want my mommy."* She was in tears and cried the phrase out repeatedly in obvious distress over the situation. I have since chalked this one up to either the work of the evil one or my long repressed emotions that must somehow find freedom whether consciously or unconsciously.

I have slowly come to understand two things quite clearly. The pain of Kelsey's death will never completely diminish. Her illness and death will always be a part of each of us as individual family members. It will also continue to be a defining characteristic of our family. The response to her death has prompted changes in each of us. As I consider those changes, I am convinced, based upon dialog with my wife and our children, that they are all positive in one way or another. Yes it still hurts. Yes we wish she were still here with us and will undoubtedly miss her until we are reunited. However, our lives go on and we live them with greater clarity, greater understanding, and greater thankfulness than we otherwise would have. I believe that because of Kelsey's life with us, and her early departure, that we all now realize the precious and fragile nature of every moment. I have never been one to verbalize my love for others, including family members. I am still woefully negligent in this area, but because of Kelsey's example, I do it more frequently than I ever did before her death. I hug more frequently as well. I am less pretentious and far less consumed with my own professional advancement and status. I count every single material possession as a gift from God that could slip through my hands and disappear in a heartbeat. And amazingly, short of some personal discomfort, I now understand that I would be none the worse for their absence. It is quite clear to me that I will leave this world with nothing including this shell of a body. I am also quite clear in my understanding, that we are all ultimately terminal in this life. It will end for all of us whether we choose to consider this reality or not. Most of us live as if we will not die. I did, and sometimes still do. The difference for me now however, is that Kelsey's death is the burr in my saddle that prompts me to remember the sheer insanity of this type of avoidance. Amazingly as well, there is also now a certain sense of joy and expectation that I experience when considering the reality of being reunited with Kelsey and other deeply loved friends and family members. Not only will we be reunited, but we will all come together in a world of perfection that will far surpass any of the wonderful times that I have enjoyed in this world with my family and friends. A world of total, complete, and uninterrupted joy; a world of wholeness and perfection; a world of total fulfillment in the work that God will have us doing; a world minus death and loss. God's world, not Satan's. This world belongs to the evil one. The next will belong to the King and His right hand man. The war will end and Jesus will use Satan and death as His footstool. Kelsey, my wife Suzanne, my son John and my daughter Katie, along with a host of friends and family will once again come together in one giant eternal celebration.

Kelsey, we're coming baby.

Until then, we will choose to cherish those we love in this world just as you did. **See you shortly!**

16

FROM DARKNESS TO LIGHT

"Was Du erlebst, kann keine Macht der Welt Dir rauben."

"What you have experienced, no power on earth can take from you." Victor Frankl

"Das, was mich nicht töten wird macht mich starker."

"That which does not kill me makes me stronger."

Friedrich Nietzsche

As I sat in my library recently, reading and alternately entertaining thoughts of the physical blessings that I observed all around me, I reached a startling conclusion. Thinking back through the years that I had struggled through college and early adulthood, I began to remember specific times and events. The nature of the events that I recalled, were a bit incongruous with the "things" that now surrounded me. Wealth is always relative, but by the standards of the world, I have become "wealthy" in regards to material possessions. I am surrounded by things. I have a wonderful house on an acre of land, two newer cars, and the biggest concerns that I have center around when we will have the cash in hand to replace worn out carpet and laminate countertops. On this day however, the events that were important to me, and were forever etched upon my heart, had nothing to do with wealth or material possessions. In fact, they were memories of times when my life was trying and difficult. The early years of my marriage for instance. Difficult, but wonderfully blessed times of learning and growing together with the woman that I have come to value more than any other through the passing years. Moving together to a new city a thousand miles from home, and as far as we were concerned,

a city that was a thousand miles from nowhere. Two long winters of zero to fifty below, and ten foot snow drifts. Two first years of marriage filled with board games together on Sunday afternoons during the worst of the winter weather. Two first years of marriage filled with "make or break" moments that we somehow managed to emerge from in one piece as well as on the "still married" side. Years spent together raising young children who couldn't understand why we bought "store brand" cereal and ate scrambled eggs for dinner. Days with sick children, two jobs, barely making ends meet and little time for each other. Difficult times for sure, but times that remain with grace and beauty in my memory, and that I treasure in my heart still today.

As I left those thoughts and continued with my reading, I was struck by the powerful message in Victor Frankl's seminal work, "Man's Search for Meaning." Having been taken by the Nazis, along with every member of his family to the Auschwitz concentration camp, he recounts the atrocities that he experienced as a result. The absolutely astonishing realization however, the construct of his experience that touched me in a powerful and profound way, was not the depravity and utter hopelessness of his situation. As far as the prisoners

knew they would never leave the camp, and their incarceration would mark the end of their existence. The exact timing and method for their death, was inexorably tied to the whims of the prison guards. The nature and impact of their plight is reflected in the following excerpts:

"When the layers of subcutaneous fat had vanished, and we looked like skeletons disguised with skin and rags, we could watch our bodies beginning to devour themselves. The organism digested its own protein, and the muscles disappeared... One after another the members of the little community in our hut died."

"One morning I heard someone, whom I knew to be brave and dignified, cry like a child because he finally had to go to the snowy marching grounds in his bare feet, as his shoes were too shrunken for him to wear."

Most certainly, these were horrible, demeaning, and frightening circumstances. Knowing daily, that a full ninety percent of their fellow prisoners would eventually find death through starvation, disease, or the gas chambers and crematoriums must have been emotionally excruciating. Knowing each morning

that some prisoners would surely die that day and not knowing whether you would die with them must have been overwhelmingly depressing, and emotionally debilitating. This is a life situation that most of us cannot even conceptualize, much less relate to.

Then I grasped the meaning of the greatest secret that human poetry and human thought and belief have to impart: The salvation of man is through love and in love. I understood how a man who has nothing left in this world still may know bliss, be it only for a brief moment, in the contemplation of his beloved."

Is it possible to experience bliss in the midst of starvation, disease and imminent death?

How is this so?

"Had I known then that my wife was dead, I think that I would still have given myself, undisturbed by that knowledge, to the contemplation of her image, and that my mental conversation with her would have been just as vivid and just as satisfying."

"Set me like a seal upon thy heart, love is as strong as death."

Now go back and reread the last two excerpts. Read them as many times as it takes to realize their full impact. Most of the prisoners who were not yet dead, eventually and understandably gave up. They simply gave their thoughts up to the past, would not rise from their cots, and allowed their bodies to deteriorate along with their outlook. Very few were able like Frankl, to establish a thought life that established meaning even in their present dehumanized condition. Frankl established meaning in the midst of his pain and suffering. At some point, whether he lived or died was of no consequence, and the meaning lay simply in his endurance of suffering and loss, and his choice to die with dignity at the same time reaching out to touch others in a powerful and positive way. In the matter of his wife, whether she remained alive or dead was inconsequential to the image that he held, and the love that he continued to entertain for her. That love remained undiminished in spite of her death.

"Set me like a seal upon thy heart, love is as strong as death."

My love for Kelsey has not diminished since her death, and I am quite sure that it never will. The

simple Biblical truth is that love always trumps death. In fact, this trump card beats every other card in the deck. There is nothing in your life that can supersede, mitigate, or overshadow love, including death. Satan desires to have you become bitter with the belief that God's love was somewhere in hiding when your loss occurred; that God somehow forgot, or didn't care enough to save your marriage, home, husband, wife, child – fill in your own blank. He would also have you believe that there was no meaning in the loss or your subsequent suffering as a result. Don't believe it. We will always maintain the ability to construct meaning from our losses and our suffering. By God's own design, between stimulus and response there is always a choice. Whether we recognize it or not, our response to the loss that we have experienced and the ensuing suffering that it invokes is a choice. Finding meaning in the loss is a choice. We make a choice to forego bitterness, and begin the hard work of finding our own personal meaning to the loss and the suffering that inevitably follows it.

During the final hours of Kelsey's life, I was shocked and offended when a pastor counseled me to give up hope for her healing. My response to this

pastor was that I had everything to gain and nothing to lose by believing that God could and would heal Kelsey. Did Kelsey's death bring hurt and suffering to my life? Of course it did. To alter and further personalize the quotation that heads this chapter:

"What I have experienced since Kelsey's death, no power on earth can take from me." The ensuing loss and suffering following Kelsey's death are mine to do with as I please. No one can take them from me, and I would surprisingly choose to not relinquish them. The same pastor also counseled me following a conversation surrounding my search to establish some type of meaning in Kelsey's death, in the following way:

John: *"I am convinced that God can direct me to a purpose or meaning to be found in Kelsey's death. I just believe that something important and powerful can result from this, I am continuing to pray for direction in finding or creating it."*

Pastor: *I understand. It makes you feel better about Kelsey's death to try and attach some meaning to it. Unfortunately, you may have to accept the fact that there may be no meaning. Sometimes these things just happen.*

What I believe this pastor and many others fail to understand is that God may allow random catastrophic loss to occur in our lives, but He has also given us the freedom in our response to the loss. One response is to establish meaning, and I believe that every loss lends itself to that possibility. Ultimately, our choices will determine our eternal destiny. We are not helpless and hapless victims in the face of a God who allows random suffering. We are beings of dignity and infinite worth to our maker, and we have been endowed with the ability to choose our response not only to Him, but to the events that occur in our lives. These events may involve great pleasure or great pain, but our choices remain the same.

Laminate or granite? Carpet or tile?

Right now I don't give a rip. My joy resides within me not without. It abides there through the power of the Holy Spirit of God, and cannot be taken away. Whether you personally believe or not has no relevance to my belief or my joy. Argue and complain if you must, but my belief will not be impacted by your struggle. We must all work out our own salvation with fear and trembling, and I

will do everything possible to aid you in your struggle. But do it for you I cannot.

My destiny is a destination where carpet and tile are utterly unimportant. They are fortuitously and completely irrelevant.

Thank God!

And God forgive me for becoming so involved in this temporary residence that I believe at times that this is all there is.

17

THE SEED OF HOPE

I was recently involved in a spiritual conversation with a young man in his early twenties. He considers himself to be an agnostic. His beliefs of course, trouble me. This is a young man with a soul that I felt may "need saving." Of course, I believed that I could facilitate the saving piece of this, based on my extensive life experience and my powerful and all encompassing grasp of all **things spiritual. This is an** engaging young man who to his

misfortune is the same age as my son. During the course of our conversations together, and my attempts to convince him that there is a wonderful God available to fill our every need if we will but ask, I discovered that like so many, he had suffered tremendous spiritual and emotional pain at the hands of a spiritually clueless pastor. It is amazing, isn't it, how many times we are hurt, and often alienated from the God we want so desperately to know, by members of the religious community? I do not know the specifics of the hurt, other than the belief that it involved this young man's non-fulfillment of a religious contract. You do know what I mean by religious contract don't you? Regardless of the terminology, we probably all understand that most churches maintain a list of doctrines that when not fulfilled, result in reprimand, and if not immediate, eventual eternal damnation to hell's burning cauldron. These doctrines are of course, our attempt to quantify religion and what we believe are spiritual values, to the extent that we can feel a sense of accomplishment and spiritual superiority as we cross each off our list of requirements for salvation. Many of these doctrines strangely mirror the Ten Commandments in an updated sort of way.

We know that we are not supposed to commit murder, and consequently, don't we feel so superior to those who have actually done what most of us consider the unthinkable act of putting an end to the life of another human being? That's a no-brainer, and we feel so good about ourselves each time we think of it and mentally cross it from our doctrinal list. Wow, I must be so much better than the guy who murdered his ex-wife! And guess what? I'm not a drug addict. Whew! Man I'm becoming more spiritual by the day! And you know what? I have never had sex with anyone but my wife – well, while we were married of course. There was that pretty dark haired girl back in college; I believe her name was Cindy. Oh yea; there were several more in my early twenties. Goodness gracious, they were all gorgeous! But I've changed since then and can now cross infidelity and promiscuity off my list. Have you ever had someone say to you from the pulpit or even in conversation that they have never had sex outside of marriage? This is a wonderful thing, but many times it is stated through the veil of moral superiority. Why would I really care whether you have or haven't? Aside from the educational value of such knowledge, I am interested in who you are now. Oh, and by the way, I'm not stealing from my

company. Goodness! I'm a better person that I thought I was!

And so the story goes…

But back to the young man; who expressed to me through eyes that were clear and bright, but seemed to belie a hidden sadness, that subsequent to the spiritual derailing that he had experienced, he worked hard at seeking and finding God with the expectation that God would heal all of his wounds through the power of His Son. He worked and worked and prayed and prayed, and from his perspective, God didn't do His part. He did not swoop into this young man's life and fix all of his hurt and pain. In fact, he kept after it for two years, and still the hole in his heart remained. He then determined that God was not who he said He was. If He were, his brokenness would have been "fixed" by now. I found myself at a complete loss when it came to a response. So I continued to listen. And I continued to relate the tremendous impact that God had on my own life through the power of the Holy Spirit. I felt compelled to intimate that the Bible was clear that Jesus was the one and only way to God which I continue to believe deeply. He does not. In the days following this conversation, I spent time in prayer and contemplation in a vain attempt to build an adequate response to his dilemma. During the course of my contemplation it became painfully clear to me that God had not as yet filled the "hole" in my own life. There continue to be days in my life that I am depressed and discouraged. As much as I ask God to complete me and take care of these issues; to "fill the hole" so to speak, he seems to sometimes leave me hanging. As I recently continued my reading of Donald Miller's new book, A Million Miles in a Thousand Years, it became increasingly clear to me that God has never promised any of us that He would fill the holes that are invariably blasted, as if by a shotgun, into our lives here on earth. In many cases, these holes are created through catastrophic loss. Miller echoes Frankl and Peck in a more modern way, *"There is a lot of money and power to be had in convincing people we can create an Eden here on earth. Cults are formed when leaders make such absurd promises. Products are sold convincing people that they are missing out on the perfect life. We all get worked into a frenzy over things that will not happen until Jesus returns. …I've got to let go of the idea that things will ever be made perfect, at least while I'm walking around on this planet."*

It's hope man! It's hope! Hope that God will make things better, indeed perfect, in another life. It is hope first and foremost, in this "other life." As M. Scott Peck states in the first chapter of The Road Less Traveled, *"Life is difficult."* Indeed it is! And it will continue to be. It is amazing however, how wonderful this life can be, when we come to the point of belief in a better world parallel with the understanding that this life will always be difficult. Not necessarily difficult on a daily basis, although the Biblical truth is that *"each day has enough difficulties of its own."* In and around those difficulties however, is unadulterated joy when we accept and experience the hope that has been placed in our hearts by an unseen hand. I now understand, that my responsibility to the young man with whom we began this chapter, is to live out the fruits of the spirit; to allow him to glimpse the pain that I have experienced, but to more clearly see the hope that I posses. I will never fully recover from my loss in this lifetime. I will never fully regain what I have lost here on this earth. Nor will you. Write it down, come back and revisit it. It is simply the way things are. Why? I haven't a clue.

If you figure it out, please email or call. I'd love to know.

18

DREAMS

Last night I dreamed that I was naked in a public place. Doubtless, many of you have had the same dream. I tend to believe that my dream indicates that I am concerned about being exposed and judged through the "baring of my soul." So be it. As I have written through my experiences with pain and loss, I have certainly "bared my soul" throughout the process. It has, to say the least, been difficult. It runs counter to my natural instinct, and is certainly not reflective of the stoic, always in control, emotionally reserved individual that I had grown to be before my daughter's diagnosis. Many times in the words of Jo Dee Mecina, I felt that I had

"been to hell on my knees and come face to face with the devil."

I have no doubt that many of you have felt the same. Witnessing my daughter sitting in our car in a stupor, covered in vomit, unable to communicate, and realizing that she was quickly fading away from us, was one of those times. It was horrible and I felt helpless. But as the song continues, "though it's hard to believe, it gets better." And you have my unconditional assurance that it does.

"I'll turn conventional wisdom on its head. I'll expose so-called experts as crackpots. Since the world in all its fancy wisdom never had a clue when it came to knowing God, God in his wisdom took delight in using what the world considered foolish…to bring those who trust him into the way of salvation." I Corinthians 1:20-21.

If you're looking for a step by step program that will lead you to healing, I can't help you. It may

work for some, but it has not for me. There has
been much pain and much trembling on the road to
recovery. I doubt that I will ever attain a full
recovery, but I assure you once again, that it does
get better. God is good, and in spite of the fact that
rotten things happen to us in this life, good things
happen as well. The beauty that I've found in the
big picture of my life, is the God given ability to
"treasure in my heart" the memories of the people,
times, places, thoughts, and feelings that I have
been given to experience during my time here..
Mary did. Her son Jesus suffered horribly before he
died. Mary watched; Mary cried; Mary felt agony
and pain for the son she loved dearly. The son she
raised from infancy to adulthood, sharing love and
memories with him through the years of his life
here on earth.

*"This child is destined to cause many in Israel
to fall, but he will be a joy to many others. He
has been sent as a sign from God, but many will
oppose him. As a result, the deepest thoughts
of many hearts will be revealed. And a sword
will pierce your very soul."* Luke 2:34-35

*"So he went back to Nazareth with them, and
lived obediently with them. And his mother*

held these things dearly and deeply within her heart." Luke 2:51

Mary has just been told that as a result of Jesus' ministry, many will oppose him and that she herself will suffer for him as if a sword has pierced her very soul. As a parent, in the face of your child's suffering, would you not feel the same "piercing of your soul?" So what does she do?

She treasures in her heart the things he says, his obedience, and their time together. When the tragedy strikes and she chooses to watch her son humiliated, tortured and murdered, what does she have left and what will she do?

Mary chooses to call back out the memories and the love that she has held deeply within her heart for all these years. This is the essence of the joy that I believe Mary was able to experience in spite of the suffering that she shared with her son.

As I continue to grapple with the intricacies and dichotomies of human existence, one thing has become clear to me, and it is simply this: As God created *spiritual* as well as *human* beings, we have been given freedom. In many cases this freedom is indeed limited, but none the less, we embody that freedom however limited it may be. There are no easy answers. Catastrophic loss is personal. The pain we feel and our reaction to the pain is unique to each of us, and God allows each of us to "work out our own salvation with fear and trembling." I have certainly experienced my share of fear and trembling. I have also experienced tremendous grace and redemption resulting from my considerable guilt. Were it not for the willingness of God's son to step into the fire of pain and death, and the willingness of His father to purposely suffer catastrophic loss through the horrendous death of his Son, I would not be relieved of that guilt, nor would I be able to face and make responsible choices regarding my own intensely painful and personal suffering. There was, is, and will continue to be, meaning in Kelsey's death. My responsibility lies in continuing to allow God to shine His light on that meaning for the benefit of others. If in some way this has been of benefit to you, I am happy! If there are other ways that my wife Suzanne and I can continue to offer help or support to you, your church, or your support group, please feel free to contact us. We would love to speak to your church or your group. We would love to help you establish a support group. We would love to speak with you

individually and listen to your story of loss, and offer support and encouragement. Our pain is unique, but our suffering can be shared.

EPILOGUE

Poets say science takes away from the beauty of the stars — mere globs of gas atoms. Nothing is 'mere'. I too can see the stars on a desert night, and feel them. But do I see less or more? The vastness of the heavens stretches my imagination — stuck on this carousel my little eye can catch one-million-year-old light. A vast pattern — of which I am a part... What is the pattern or the meaning or the why? It does not do harm to the mystery to know a little more about it. ~ Richard Feynman

I have heard it said that as human beings we are not even sure that we consist of solid material. Just like a table or a chair, we consist of an amalgamation of molecules, which consist of an amalgamation of atoms, which in turn consist of an amalgamation of sub atomic particles. In the end, at the most miniscule level, our bodies consist of the tiniest of particles none of which is completely solid in and of itself. We are not our bodies. We are something infinitely more. Something that we can only attempt to grasp, but that deep, deep down we know exist. Our existence is

infinite and ultimately non-physical. Our bodies are
nothing but shells to house the most beautiful of
God's creations. On the exterior they are deceptively
simple yet inside they are incredibly complex; The
image of an invisible God, that is now visible only to
Him. We have a seed planted within us that allows us
to sense this essence in ourselves and others. It is an
essence that exists far beyond the flesh and blood that
we now see. One day without doubt, there will be a
new and eternal body to house this nature that has
been created in the image of the Creator. We can only
guess at what they will be and how they will look. My
belief is that they will be a perfect representation of
the very essence of each of us; the essence that we
can now only sense. I for one, will make every effort
to see beyond the physical; to sense as it were, the
essence that goes far beyond the physical to define
each of us as we truly are; the very core of our being.
This is the Kelsey that I will recognize when we are
together again.

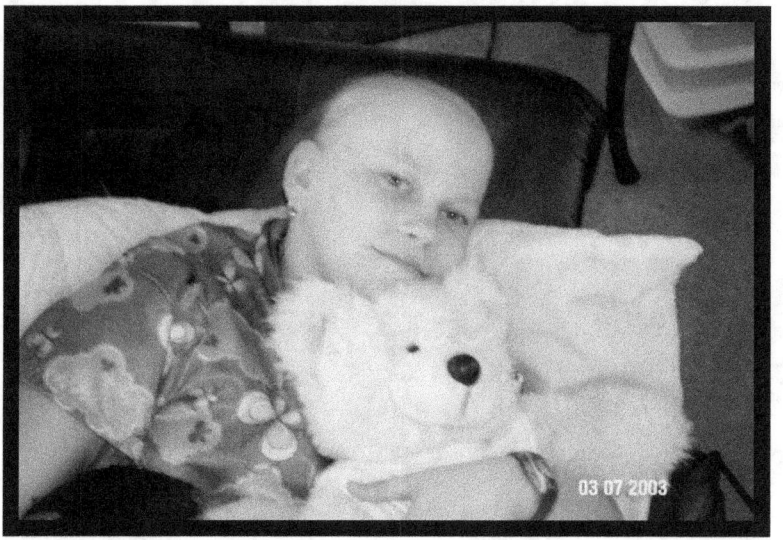

Visit us on the website at:

lifeliesbook.org

Email us at:

help@lifeliesbook.org